The *International Journal of Behavioral Medicine* is the Official Journal of the International Society of Behavioral Medicine. Member societies are the Academy of Behavioral Medicine Research (USA), American Psychosomatic Society, Australian Society of Behavioral Medicine and Health, Behavioral Medicine Section of the Czech Medical Association, Behavioral Medicine Section of the Finnish Association of Social Medicine, Danish Society of Psychosocial Medicine, French Society of Behavioral Medicine, German Society of Behavioral Medicine and Behavior Modification, Hungarian Society of Behavioural Sciences and Medicine, Japanese Society of Behavioral Medicine, Netherlands Behavioral Medicine Federation, Norwegian Society of Behavioral Medicine, Psychosomatic and Behavioral Medicine Section of the Slovak Medical Society, Slovak Society of Psychosomatic and Behavioral Medicine, Society of Behavioral Medicine (USA), Swedish Society of Behavioral Medicine, Thai Society of Behavioral Medicine, and Venezuelan Interdisciplinary Group of Behavioral Medicine. The Division of Health Psychology of the American Psychological Association, Health Psychology Section of the Canadian Psychological Association, Society of Pediatric Psychology (USA), and Special Group in Health Psychology of the British Psychological Society are affiliate members.

First published 2002 by Lawrence Erlbaum Associates, Inc.

Published 2016 by Routledge
2 Park Square, Milton Park, Abingdon, Oxon OX14 4RN
711 Third Avenue, New York, NY 10017, USA

Routledge is an imprint of the Taylor & Francis Group, an informa business

This journal is abstracted or indexed in *Focus on: Index Medicus/MEDLINE; Clinical & Treatment Research; ISI: Current Contents/Social & Behavioral Sciences; Research Alert; Social Sciences Citation Index; Social SciSearch.* Microform copies of this journal are available through ProQuest Information and Learning, P.O. Box 1346 Ann Arbor, MI 48106-1346 For more information call 1-800-521-0600 x 2888 For more information, call 1-800-521-0600 x2888.

ISBN 13: 978-0-8058-9647-3 (pbk)

INTERNATIONAL JOURNAL OF
BEHAVIORAL MEDICINE

Volume 9, Number 3

2002

Special Issue:
on
Women's Health

INTERNATIONAL JOURNAL OF BEHAVIORAL MEDICINE, 9(3), 173–175
Copyright © 2002, Lawrence Erlbaum Associates, Inc.

EDITORIAL

New Directions in Understanding the Link Between Stress and Health in Women

Historically, women have been underrepresented in health research. The focus was disproportionately on men because of concerns about the excess premature mortality in men, the changing hormone levels in women that could confound study results, and the possibility of pregnancy in women during clinical trials. Health research in women was limited to studies of diseases affecting fertility and reproduction. In response to the dearth of information, investigators have increasingly devoted their talents to identifying unique issues relevant to women's health. This special issue on women's health for the *International Journal of Behavioral Medicine* is the beneficiary of these efforts. The articles herein represent, in our minds, some of the newest directions that are being taken in behavioral medicine research on women's health.

Perhaps the most important trend evident in the seven articles in this special issue is the emphasis on the role of the social environment in determining stress, health, and well-being. Psychosocial factors involve both the "*psych*" side (i.e., psychological variables such as emotion, cognition, and personality) and the "*social*" side (i.e., social support, social roles, and social class). Historically, the "*psych*" factors have been predominant in our models. There are numerous studies, for example, of the impact of such risk factors as hostility, anger, depression, and anxiety on a variety of physical health endpoints. More recently, however, there has been considerable interest in the social stressors that trigger these stress responses and ultimately translate into health or disease.

Such a shift is evident in this special issue. Of the seven articles, four focus on gender-relevant social stressors and their impact on health. The article by Mishra, Ball, Dobson, Byles, and Warner-Smith, for example, calls for a gender-specific conceptualization and operationalization of socioeconomic status (SES). Although SES is a powerful determinant of health and well-being, it is possible that for women, traditional measures of SES are imprecise markers of social status. Some investigators infer SES in women from the SES of their husbands. But how do we assess SES in unmarried women? If we were able to identify measures of SES that worked equally as well in married and unmarried women, it is possible that we would have a powerful tool for identifying how the social environment exerts an impact on women's health. This article raises these questions and presents an approach for assessing SES that is valid across two national surveys of women living in Australia.

Two of the articles in this special issue focus on the impact of women's roles on health. As the Lee and Powers article argues, the number of social roles that a woman has could work for or against her. It could work for her if these roles provide informational and emotional support and feelings of control and self-worth (the enhancement hypothesis). It could work against her if these roles present competing demands that are difficult to reconcile (the scarcity hypothesis). These researchers hypothesize that the impact of multiple roles on women varies by age. Drawing on a large survey of Australian women, they provide data to support this hypothesis and show further that the greatest risk for chronic disease and lower quality of life is for those women, at any age, who have no roles.

The other article on social roles, by King, Atienza, Castro, and Collins, takes a closer look at caregiving—a role that is increasing in importance with the progressive aging of our population. These researchers used ambulatory monitoring to study hemodynamic responses to caring for a demented relative. They compared responses of wives to those of daughters and found that the daughters fared more poorly in the face of this stressor. This is a disturbing observation when one considers the demographic transition that is occurring where larger numbers of elderly people are living with greater levels of disability. We simply must find ways to keep the caregivers healthy.

It is well accepted that women enjoy as much or more social support than do men, but actually derive less physical health benefits from it. The article by Uno, Uchino, and Smith takes a closer look at the nature of support in women and suggests that support may provide a buffer against heightened cardiovascular responses to psychological stress only if it is provided in a high-quality relationship. Social support provided in relationships characterized by ambivalence actually may have an adverse impact on health outcomes.

One of the articles in this special issue focuses on a unique potential physiological mechanism by which chronic stress translates into a health outcome. Anderson and Chesney propose the hypothesis that chronic stress links to hypertension through the mechanism of *inhibited* breathing. This, at first glance, is counterintuitive because emotional arousal is more commonly associated with increased sympathetic nervous system activation and, as such, *increased* breathing. The researchers suggest, however, that relaxed breathing and subnormal breathing are often confused. They go on to demonstrate that those who experience high perceived stress over the prior month have more inhibited breathing. They find this stress and breathing link to be particularly pronounced for women. A highlight of this article is the integrated and systematic program of research that these investigators are pursuing and the importance of this particular article to their understanding of the moderating effects of gender on it.

The final two articles have implications for interventions with women. The first used cluster analytic techniques, and found that women were more likely than men to link their somatic problems to stress, particularly excessive work demands. Because they are more likely to identify stress as a causal factor for health, they may be more willing to undergo interventions to reduce stress as a way to improve health.

The Burrell and Granlund article, however, sounds an alarm about our past record of success in interventions for women. Focusing on the subgroup of women with coronary disease, these researchers point to the importance of *not* generalizing to women the results of interventions that have been effective for men. The most recent clinical trials of psychosocial factors in post-myocardial infarction patients, including The Montreal Heart Attack Readjustment Trial (MHART) and The Enhancing Recovery in Coronary Heart Disease Patients Trial (ENRICHD), actually showed that the psychosocial intervention might have harmed some women on the major clinical endpoints. This challenges our popular assumption that we will do no harm, but might do some good. It is possible that a psychosocial intervention could do some harm. This suggests caution in taking the next steps in this line of research. We believe, as do Burrell and Granlund, that it is time to take a step back and to start listening to women, understanding their unique problems, and developing interventions that are responsive to these concerns. Starting small with pilot work and building up to more ambitious studies may be the best way to guard against the possibility of doing harm. A highlight of the Burrell and Granlund article is that they provide us with their clinical insights, derived from years of working with female coronary patients. They go on to translate these insights into a description of a pilot intervention study that is tailored specifically to the concerns of women with coronary disease.

In summary, the articles included in this special issue on women's health suggest some new directions in behavioral medicine research on women. We are seeing more sophisticated models of the link between stress and disease. Earlier models that documented the pathways between stress and disease are being replaced with newer models that document the pathways from social stressors to psychobiological responses and ultimately to health and disease. It is clear that the social stressors that trigger the stress response differ between men and women. It is exciting to see research that begins to identify unique stressors for women, including absence of meaningful roles, caregiving, and ambiguous social relationships. An equally important direction is to begin to translate results from the sophisticated observational studies into efficacious and effective interventions. In this line of research, we may need to take a step back before taking a step forward.

Lynda H. Powell
Karen A. Matthews

INTERNATIONAL JOURNAL OF BEHAVIORAL MEDICINE, 9(3), 176–194

Physiological and Affective Responses to Family Caregiving in the Natural Setting in Wives Versus Daughters

Abby C. King, Audie Atienza,
Cynthia Castro and Rakale Collins

This study examined differences in hemodynamic responses to usual caregiving duties undertaken in the natural setting by caregiving wives versus daughters. Participants were 88 women (36 daughters, 52 wives), 50 years of age or older, caring for a relative with dementia. Participants underwent 2 standard laboratory challenges (1 physical and 1 emotional) and ambulatory monitoring in the natural setting. Although wives and daughters showed similar physiological responses to the laboratory challenges, daughters evidenced greater hemodynamic responses in the natural setting relative to wives when the care recipient was present ($p < .02$). The increases in hemodynamic responses were accompanied by increased negative interactions with the care recipient as well as other family members ($p < .0009$). The results add to the small body of research indicating that family caregiving may have negative acute effects on psychosocial and physiological responses in the natural setting, particularly in daughters.

Abby C. King, Division of Epidemiology, Department of Health Research & Policy, and Stanford Center for Research in Disease Prevention, Department of Medicine, Stanford University School of Medicine, CA, USA. Audie Atienza, Stanford Center for Research in Disease Prevention, Department of Medicine, Stanford University School of Medicine, CA, USA. Cynthia Castro, Stanford Center for Research in Disease Prevention, Department of Medicine, Stanford University School of Medicine; and Rakale Collins, Social Epidemiology Research Division, Morehouse School of Medicine, Atlanta, GA, USA.

This research was funded by PHS Grant AG–12358 from the National Institute on Aging awarded to Dr. King and PHS–NHLBI Training Grant 5T32HL07034 awarded to Stephen P. Fortmann. We gratefully acknowledge the help and assistance provided by Kellie Baumann and Paula O'Sullivan in participant recruitment and data collection activities and by David Ahn in data analysis.

Correspondence concerning this article should be addressed to Abby C. King, Stanford Center for Research in Disease Prevention, Stanford University School of Medicine, 730 Welch Road, Suite B, Palo Alto, CA 94304–1583.

Key words: family caregiving, hemodynamic responses, ambulatory monitoring

Providing informal care to an infirm or disabled older family member on a regular basis (i.e., family caregiving) has become an increasingly prevalent life role for middle- and older-aged women in the United States as well as other industrialized nations (Lee & Porteous, 1998; National Alliance for Caregiving and the American Association of Retired Persons, 1997; Stone, Cafferata, & Sangl, 1987). Iatrogenic physical, psychological, social, and financial effects of the caregiving role have been increasingly documented (Russo, Vitaliano, Brewer, Katon, & Becker, 1995; Schulz & Beach, 1999; Schulz, O'Brien, Bookwala, & Fleissner, 1995) and appear to be exacerbated when the care recipient is suffering from dementia (Goode, Haley, Roth, & Ford, 1998; Ory, Hofffman, Yee, Tennstedt, & Schulz, 1999; Schulz et al., 1995). Among the detrimental health effects of family caregiving among at least some groups of older caregivers are an increased vulnerability to physical illness (Stone et al., 1987), as well as disruptions in immune function (Kiecolt-Glaser, Marucha, Malarkey, & al., 1995; Wu et al., 1999) and metabolic regulation (Vitaliano, Scanlan, Siegler, McCormick, & Knopp, 1998). The potentially devastating impact of such physical perturbations on the health of family caregivers has been underscored recently by the Caregiver Health Study, in which family caregiving accompanied by emotional strain was an independent risk factor for mortality among older adults (Schulz & Beach, 1999).

Virtually all of these studies have focused on physical health outcomes in response to the chronic effects of the caregiving experience. Investigation of the more immediate, *acute* physiological effects of caregiving on stress-responsive pathways that may, over time, generate or exacerbate disease processes has received minimal attention (Mills, Yi, Ziegler, Patterson, & Grant, 1999; Vitaliano, Russo, Bailey, Young, & McCann, 1993). One such pathway potentially mediating the relation between stress and cardiovascular morbidity and mortality outcomes in caregivers is cardiovascular responsivity to stress (Kral et al., 1997). One study evaluated the acute effects of the caregiving experience on blood pressure (BP) and heart rate (HR) responses throughout the day, measured via ambulatory monitoring in the caregiver's natural setting (King, Oka, & Young, 1994). The results indicated that although caregivers and noncaregivers showed comparable hemodynamic responses in clinical and work settings, caregivers demonstrated a significant increase in BP levels, relative to noncaregivers, following work, particularly when they were in the presence of the care recipient (King et al., 1994).

The majority of family care for older adults with dementia is carried out by either wives or daughters (National Alliance for Caregiving and the American Association of Retired Persons, 1997; Stone et al., 1987). In light of the differing relationship as well as challenges occurring when the care recipient is one's spouse as opposed to one's parent (Skaff & Pearlin, 1992), much of the caregiving literature is comprised of studies focusing on either spousal caregivers (Vitaliano, Dougherty, & Siegler, 1994; Vitaliano, Russo, Young, Teri, & Maiuro, 1991; Wu et al., 1999) or daughters (Christensen, Stephens, & Townsend, 1998; Stephens & Townsend, 1997). For example, the previously described study of hemodynamic responses to caregiving in the natural environment included only daughters (King et al., 1994). Yet, the inclusion of both wives and daughters provides an opportunity to gain a greater understanding of the differential effects of family caregiving for these two important caregiver subgroups (Alspaugh, Stephens, Townsend, Zarit, & Greene, 1999; Li, Seltzer, & Greenberg, 1997; Skaff & Pearlin, 1992; Strawbridge, Wallhagen, Shemea, & Kaplan, 1997; Young & Kahana, 1989).

The goal of this investigation was to evaluate hemodynamic responses to the usual caregiving duties undertaken in the natural setting in caregiving wives versus daughters. In light of the greater potential for role conflicts that could adversely affect physiological responses among child, relative to spousal, caregivers (Skaff & Pearlin, 1992; Strawbridge et al., 1997; Young & Kahana, 1989), we hypothesized that daughters would evidence more elevated hemodynamic responses to their caregiving situation relative to wives. In addition, we explored psychosocial and behavioral correlates of the hemodynamic responses observed in the natural setting.

METHOD

Participants

Participants were 88 women (36 daughters and 52 wives) who had enrolled in the Teaching Healthy Lifestyles for Caregivers study. Eligibility criteria for the major trial were: postmenopausal, 50 years of age or older (could be 46 to 49 years if participant was postmenopausal due to a complete hysterectomy), a woman caregiver (defined as caring for a relative with Alzheimer's disease or another form of dementia, as documented by the care recipient's physician, in the caregiver's home), providing as least 10 hr of unpaid care per week, free from any medical conditions or disorders that would limit participation in light to moderate intensity exercise (e.g., walking), not participating in a regular program of physical activity (i.e., less than 3 times per week of exercise lasting 20 min or more per session over the past 6 months), and stable on all medications for at least 3 months prior to study entry.

Procedure

Recruitment occurred via community-wide promotion, including use of an array of media sources as well as referrals from physicians and organizations serving older adults and caregivers (Wilcox & King, 1999). Each participant attended two base-line assessment visits, generally occurring within a 2-week period, at the Stanford University Clinical Research Facility. Eligible participants were subsequently ran-domized into a 1-year health intervention program (nutrition or exercise). Data pre-sented in this investigation are from the baseline testing that occurred prior to ran-domization.

Measures

Demographics.   Participants completed a measure of demographic charac-teristics, including their age (in years), marital status, ethnicity, education (in years), and employment status (Wilcox & King, 1999).

Caregiving characteristics.   Participants completed a survey focused on different aspects of their caregiving experience (King & Brassington, 1997). Items included their familial relationship to the care recipient, age of care recipient, diag-nosis of care recipient (confirmed by the care recipient's physicians), length of time as a caregiver (years or months), and average hours per week spent caregiving. Caregiver burden was assessed with the 25-item Screen for Caregiver Burden (Vitaliano, Russo, Young, Becker, & Maiuro, 1991).

Measurement of hemodynamic responses in a standard setting.   To evaluate whether there was a general predisposition toward higher levels of physiological responsiveness in either wives or daughters independent of set-ting, participants underwent a laboratory-based physical challenge (submaximal treadmill exercise test) and emotional challenge (interpersonal in-terview focused on their caregiving experience) prior to hemodynamic assess-ment in the natural setting. These two challenges are described later. Partici-pants were instructed to refrain from caffeine intake and cigarette smoking for at least 2 hr prior to these assessments.

Treadmill exercise test (physical challenge).   Participants performed an ECG-monitored, symptom-limited, graded treadmill exercise test using a Balke-type protocol with workloads increasing by approximately 1.0 to 2.0 meta-bolic equivalents every 2 min (American College of Sports Medicine, 1986). Prior to beginning the treadmill test, participants rested quietly in a supine position for 5 min, at the end of which pretest HR and BP levels were assessed. Submaximal HR and BP levels were determined at the end of the second 2-min stage (treadmill speed at 2 miles per hour; grade at 7.5% incline; 4.5 MET work level). The submaximal portion of the test assesses an individual's physiological response to a standard, moderate-intensity physical challenge.

Laboratory-based emotional challenge.   The laboratory-based psychological stressor, which occurred on the morning of the first assessment day, consisted of an interpersonal interview with a trained research technician that focused on negative aspects of the individual's caregiving situation. The protocol began with a 10-min rest period during which time the participant sat alone quietly in a room and listened to relaxing music via headphones (baseline). Following that period, a trained research assistant directed the participant to speak for about 6 min about the aspects of her caregiving experience that she found to be particularly frustrating or disturbing. The research assistant made minimal verbal responses during the task period. Following the 6-min task period, the research assistant left the room and the participant rested for an additional 10 min (the recovery period). HR and BP recordings were collected every 2 min from the beginning of the baseline period through the recovery period using a Colin ambulatory BP monitor (Model ABPM–630; Colin Medical Instruments, Plainfield, NJ) attached to the nondominant arm. The recordings were averaged within each portion of the emotional challenge (i.e., baseline, task, recovery) to obtain mean HR, systolic blood pressure (SBP), and diastolic blood pressure (DBP) levels. Reactivity levels were obtained by subtracting the mean baseline from mean task levels for each hemodynamic variable. Such speaking tasks involving emotionally relevant content have been shown to provide a reliable means of eliciting elevations in hemodynamic variables in a variety of populations of women (Carels, Szczepanski, Blumenthal, & Sherwood, 1998), including family caregivers (Vitaliano et al., 1993).

Ambulatory assessment of BP and HR in the natural setting.   The procedures for collection of ambulatory monitoring data have been described previously (King et al., 1994) and are briefly described here. Following the emotional challenge, the Colin Medical Instruments Model ABPM–630 ambulatory BP monitor remained attached to the nondominant arm. In studies investigating the accuracy of the Colin ABPM monitor compared to simultaneous intra-arterial BP readings, the monitor has been reported to be accurate, showing less disparity and closer limits of agreement with intra-arterial BP recordings than clinician-derived BP measurements (White, Lund-Johansen, & McCabe, 1989; White, Lund-Johansen, & Omvik, 1990). The Colin monitor records BP through use of both oscillometric and auscultatory (Korotkoff sound) methods (White et al., 1989). The oscillometric method measures BP through perception of the oscillometric waves generated by the brachial artery during cuff deflation. Because the two methods provided reasonably close readings in the study sample and more complete data were obtained through the less sound-sensitive oscillometric method, readings from this latter method are reported.

The ambulatory BP recorder was set to automatically record at hourly intervals up until the time that the participant retired for the night. The ambulatory recording portion of the protocol began in the early afternoon (i.e., around 1:00 p.m.) immediately following the participants' study assessment visit. The decision to use hourly BP recordings rather than more frequent recordings (e.g., 20- or 30-min intervals) was based on information obtained during a previous study with female caregivers (King et al., 1994). In that study, caregivers noted that recordings that occurred more frequently rather than on an hourly schedule posed undue burden. To minimize movement artifact that could interfere with BP recordings, participants were instructed to remain in the position that they were in at the initiation of cuff inflation and to minimize undue movement of the cuffed arm (White et al., 1989). The recorder was held in a waist belt, with leads to the cuff worn under clothing to minimize disruption or inconvenience.

Participants were instructed subsequently in the use of a Casio PB–1000 (Casio Corporation, Tokyo, Japan) pocket computer for the recording of psychosocial and health-related information throughout the day (King et al., 1994). The PB–1000 weighs 440 g, including batteries and RAM expansion pack, and is 2.5 cm × 19 cm × 18 cm when folded. It has a built-in clock and calendar, and a 32-column × 4-line LCD touch-sensitive screen. This pocket computer-based logging system has been used extensively by our group as well as other researchers at Stanford (Taylor, Fried, & Kenardy, 1990), and has been found to be an accurate and reliable method for obtaining information on behavioral variables in the natural environment (King et al., 1994; Taylor et al., 1990).

The participant's location (e.g., home, work, other location); position during each BP measurement (i.e., standing, sitting, lying prone); interpersonal contacts (i.e., occurrence of a negative or positive interaction along with the person with whom it occurred, e.g., care receiver, other family member, coworker, friend); physical activity levels (rated on a Likert scale); and intake of caffeine, alcohol, and medications (answered as yes/no) were recorded on an hourly basis throughout the day that coincided with the hourly inflation of the BP recorder (King et al., 1994; Taylor et al., 1990).

The pocket computer was programmed to automatically inform the participant each hour, via a series of auditory beeps, that it was time to complete the diary. Diary completion was accomplished by having the participant, through touching the computer screen, respond to the series of 22 questions that automatically flashed onto the screen at the designated time. The diary took approximately 3 min to complete. If the participant was unresponsive to the initial series of auditory signals, the microcomputer would continue the auditory signals for 10 min, after which time it would terminate the signal pattern until the next designated time for data entry arrived.

All participants were requested to wear the ambulatory monitor and complete the computerized diary from early afternoon to just before they retired for the night. The ambulatory BP recorder data were subsequently downloaded to a Nippon Colin AS–100 printer (Nippon Colin Co., Nagoya, Japan) for readout. The pocket computer diary data were downloaded to a Macintosh computer through use of a Casio MD–100A 3.5-inch floppy disk drive (Casio Corporation).

Data Analysis

Descriptive statistics, including independent-sample t tests, were conducted on the wife and daughter caregiver groups. Hypothesis-testing evaluating wife–daughter differences in hemodynamic responses in the natural setting were undertaken using a two-step approach as a means of reducing potential proliferation of Type I error. A multivariate analysis of variance (MANOVA) was used initially as an omnibus test incorporating the three hemodynamic variables. Subsequent analyses were planned for each hemodynamic variable contingent on the MANOVA reaching statistical significance. In light of the potential relation between age and BP levels that has been reported consistently in the literature, the planned analyses consisted initially of analysis of covariance procedures in which age was used as a covariate. Because results of the analyses of covariance were similar to those undertaken using independent-sample t tests, the more straightforward t-test results are presented.

Previous work evaluating ambulatory hemodynamic responses in female caregivers has indicated the importance of differentiating the time periods during the day when the caregiver was either with or not with the care recipient (King & Brassington, 1997; King et al., 1994). Given these findings, the ambulatory BP and HR data were analyzed separately for these two time periods, identified via the portable computerized diary (King & Brassington, 1997; King et al., 1994) using separate MANOVAs. Paired-comparison t tests were used to provide descriptive data on behavioral and social variables when the care recipient was either present or absent. Alpha was set at .05 (two-tailed tests).

RESULTS

Descriptive Analysis

Description of participants.   Descriptive statistics for wife and daughter caregivers are shown in Table 1. The two groups were comparable with respect to years of education, ethnicity, care recipient diagnosis, length of time caring for the family member, objective and subjective caregiver burden levels, smoking status (only one participant—a daughter—was a current smoker), percentage who were

TABLE 1
Baseline Demographic Characteristics for Wife and Daughter
Caregivers (Means ± Standard Deviations, Percentages)

Variable	Wives[a]	Daughters[b]
Age (years)[c]	67.9 ± 8.7	56.8 ± 5.4
Married (%)[d]	100.0	47.5
Education (years)	14.8 ± 2.8	15.3 ± 2.1
White (%)	92.2	85.0
Employed (%)[d]	17.7	50.0
Number of people in household[d]	2.3 ± 0.7	3.1 ± 1.3
Body mass index (kg/m²)	27.1 ± 5.1	28.3 ± 4.6
Age of care recipient (years)[c]	75.9 ± 8.5	85.0 ± 6.6
Alzheimer diagnosis (%)	59.0	67.5
Length of caregiving (years)	4.4 ± 3.4	3.5 ± 2.7
Objective burden score	11.5 ± 4.1	12.6 ± 3.8
Subjective burden score	41.7 ± 10.8	41.3 ± 8.8

[a]$n = 52$. [b]$n = 36$. [c]Wives vs. daughters different at $p < .0001$. [d]Wives versus Daughters different at $p < .002$.

taking antihypertensive medications (approximately 29% across the sample as a whole), and body mass index ($p > .10$). The objective and subjective caregiver burden levels, as well as length of time caregiving, were similar to other family caregiving populations reported in the literature (King et al., 1994; Vitaliano et al., 1993). As expected, wife caregivers were significantly older and a greater percentage was married relative to daughters ($p < .001$). Seventy three percent of daughters were caring for their mother. A significantly greater percentage of daughters were currently employed outside of the home relative to wives ($p < .001$). Daughters reported a significantly greater number of people living in their household relative to wives ($p < .002$).

Hemodynamic responses in the laboratory setting: Submaximal exercise test.   Mean HR and BP recordings taken during the submaximal treadmill exercise test are shown in Table 2. There were no significant HR or BP differences observed for wife versus daughter caregivers either at rest (i.e., pretest) or at submaximal exercise levels. Both caregiver groups showed a level of HR increase during the submaximal treadmill exercise test commensurate with that expected from a reasonably inactive sample of older women (King et al., 2000).

Hemodynamic responses in the laboratory setting: Emotional challenge.
The mean HR and BP recordings taken during the laboratory-based emotional challenge are shown in Table 2. There were no significant mean HR or BP differ-

ences observed for wife versus daughter caregivers during the initial rest (pretest) period prior to the challenge. Nor were there significant mean BP or HR differences observed for wife versus daughter caregivers either during the emotional challenge itself or during the subsequent 10- min recovery period immediately following the challenge. Both caregiver groups had task-related SBP and DBP increases of approximately 15 mmHg and 9 mmHg, respectively—response levels similar to those reported in a number of other laboratory- based reactivity studies of adult women and men (Carels et al., 1998; King, Taylor, Albright, & Haskell, 1990; Matthews et al., 1986).

In summary, no statistically significant differences were detected among wife versus daughter caregivers in mean BP and HR responses taken both at rest as well as during standard laboratory-based physical and emotional challenges.

TABLE 2
Heart Rate (HR), Systolic Blood Pressure (SBP) and Diastolic Blood Pressure (DBP) for
the Two Laboratory Challenges, by Wife Versus Daughter Caregiver Status[a]
(Means ± Standard Deviations)

Variable	Wives[d]	Daughters[e]
Physical challenge[b]		
Pre-task		
HR (beats/min)	73.3 ± 13.6	77.8 ± 10.7
SBP (mmHg)	132.7 ± 14.1	124.8 ± 16.9
DBP (mmHg)	79.9 ± 11.1	77.4 ± 8.6
Submax level		
HR (beats/min)	116.5 ± 17.9	112.6 ± 14.3
SBP (mmHg)	160.4 ± 22.9	151.1 ± 25.7
DBP (mmHg)	79.6 ± 11.2	80.4 ± 7.8
Emotional challenge[c]		
Rest		
HR (beats/min)	65.1 ± 9.1	67.6 ± 12.4
SBP (mmHg)	137.8 ± 17.3	132.0 ± 19.3
DBP (mmHg)	77.0 ± 9.0	76.1 ± 9.9
Task		
HR (beats/min)	72.1 ± 9.8	76.3 ± 10.6
SBP (mmHg)	153.7 ± 18.9	145.4 ± 18.4
DBP (mmHg)	85.2 ± 10.5	84.9 ± 10.9
Recovery		
HR (beats/min)	67.4 ± 10.0	67.9 ± 9.8
SBP (mmHg)	138.3 ± 16.8	130.5 ± 15.0
DBP (mmHg)	77.3 ± 9.1	76.7 ± 9.3

[a]All p values for analyses comparing wives and daughters > .05. [b]Treadmill exercise test. [c]Laboratory-based emotional challenge consisting of an interpersonal interview focused on the negative aspects of the individual's caregiving situation. [d]$n = 52$. [e]$n = 36$.

Hypothesis Testing Related to Hemodynamic Responses in the Natural Setting.   Wife and daughter caregivers had a similar number of hourly ambulatory BP and HR recordings in the natural setting (*M* number of recordings = 8.3 + 2.2 for wives and 8.2 + 2.4 for daughters; difference *ns*). As noted earlier, to explore the elevations in HR and DBP in the natural setting, the portable computerized diary results were used to divide the day into two time periods based on whether the care recipient was present or not (*M* number of hourly recordings during the time period when the care recipient was present = 5.6 + 2.6 for wives and 3.4 + 2.6 for daughters, difference *ns*; *M* number of recordings during the time period when the care recipient was not present = 4.3 + 2.5 for wives and 5.8 + 2.9 for daughters; difference *ns*). The MANOVA evaluating wife–daughter differences in hemodynamic responses when in the presence of the care recipient was significant, $F(3, 71) = 2.88, p < .04$. Planned independent-sample *t* tests on each hemodynamic variable indicated that daughters, relative to wives, had significantly greater DBP (*M* between-group difference = 6.7, $p < .0007$, 95% confidence interval = 2.33–10.99) and HR levels (*M* between-group difference = 5.2, $p < .02$, 95% confidence interval = 1.60–9.84) during this time period (see Figure 1). Between-group differences were not found in SBP responses during this time period.

In contrast, the MANOVA evaluating wife–daughter differences in hemodynamic responses when the care recipient was not present did not reach statistical significance ($p > .80$; see Figure 1).

Within-group analyses, undertaken for descriptive purposes, indicated that daughters had significantly greater mean SBP and DBP levels when they were in the presence of the care recipient relative to when the care recipient was absent; *M* within-group difference for SBP = 5.7 ($t = 2.4$), $p < .02$; *M* within-group difference for DBP = 5.2 ($t = 3.0$), $p < .006$. There were no significant within-group differences for wives.

Exploring Potential Confounds Influencing Wife–Daughter Hemodynamic Differences

Because of the greater percentage of daughters working outside of the home relative to wives, the period of time when daughters were in the presence of the care recipient tended to be shifted somewhat toward evening as opposed to afternoon hours. To determine whether the wife–daughter differences in BP and HR levels occurring in the presence of the care recipient were due primarily to time of day effects (i.e., afternoon vs. evening), as opposed to care recipient effects, wife–daughter ambulatory responses were compared in the afternoon and evening hours. In contrast to the significant differences found for the time period when the care recipient was present, no significant between-group differences in any of the three hemodynamic variables were found when the day was divided into the afternoon and the evening periods.

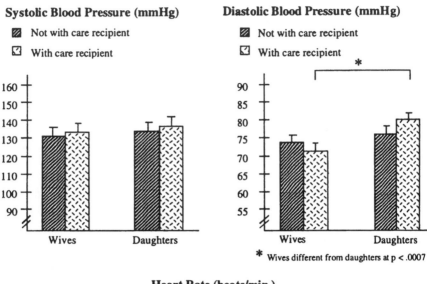

Systolic Blood Pressure (mmHg)

Diastolic Blood Pressure (mmHg)

* Wives different from daughters at p < .0007

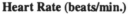

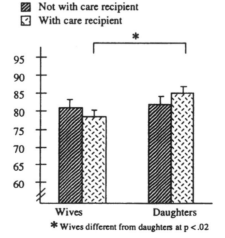

Heart Rate (beats/min.)

* Wives different from daughters at p < .02

FIGURE 1 Systolic blood pressure, diastolic blood pressure, and heart rate responses (means and standard errors) in the natural setting for wives versus daughters, when the care recipient was present versus absent.

Similarly, to evaluate the potential effects of the variables, in addition to age, on which wives and daughters differed significantly (i.e., employment status, marital status, caregiver recipient gender and age, number of people in the household), we re-ran the analyses on hemodynamic variables in the natural setting described earlier, controlling for each of these variables in turn. As with age, no significant differences were found when each of these variables was included in the model. In addition, when several of these variables were compared within the daughter group itself (i.e., t tests comparing married vs. unmarried daughters; employed versus unemployed daughters), the means for the subgroups being compared were virtually indistinguishable from one another ($p > .10$).

To ascertain whether the differences noted in ambulatory hemodynamic responses between wives and daughters could be due to differences in other relevant behavioral factors occurring during the day, results from the portable computerized diary were used to compare wives and daughters on levels of physical activity; postural position at the time of the BP/HR rate recordings; and caffeine, alcohol, or medication use throughout the day. No significant wife–daughter differences were found for any of these variables, either across the day as a whole or when the day was broken into the two time periods described earlier (i.e., care recipient present vs. absent).

Relation of Psychosocial Factors to Hemodynamic Responses in the Natural Setting

In addition to the potential impact of the aforementioned behavioral factors on hemodynamic responses in the natural setting, a growing literature has documented the potential iatrogenic effects of negative social interactions with significant others on hemodynamic responses, both in laboratory and naturalistic settings (Carels et al., 1998; Ewart & Koldner, 1991). To evaluate this variable in this investigation, the portable computerized diary data were used to identify how often throughout the day caregivers recorded the occurrence of at least one distressing verbal interaction within the hour preceding each BP/HR measurement. The occurrence of such an event, coded as either 0 (*absent*) or 1 (*present*), was then averaged across the day for each caregiver. Across the day as a whole, the mean percentage of hourly recordings containing at least one recorded distressing interaction was significantly greater for daughters (*M* percentage of hourly recordings in which at least one distressing interaction occurred = 0.62 + 0.33) relative to wives (*M* = 0.36 + 0.38; $p < .003$). When evaluated by whether the care recipient was present or absent, the wife–daughter difference in frequency of a distressing interaction was found only during that period when the caregiver was in the presence of the care recipient (*M* for daughters = 0.63 + 0.36; *M* for wives = 0.32 + 0.38, $p < .0009$, 95% confidence interval = .13 – .49). When the care recipient was absent, *M* for daughters = 0.39 + 0.42; *M* for wives =

0.31 + 0.42; *ns*. Based on the portable computerized diary information, a substantial percentage of these distressing interactions (approximately 60% for daughters and 69% for wives) were with the care recipient. For daughter caregivers, another 26% of the distressing interactions during the care recipient–present time period occurred with other family members (compared with 11% for wife caregivers).

To further evaluate the relation between hemodynamic responses and the occurrence of distressing interactions with the care recipient for wives and daughters, within-group analyses were undertaken. Specifically, for wives and daughters separately, paired-comparison *t* tests were conducted comparing each of the three hemodynamic variables in turn during the time periods when a distressing interaction was reported versus when a distressing interaction was not reported. For daughters, DBP responses were significantly higher when a distressing interaction occurred relative to when a distressing interaction was not reported (M difference in DBP across these two time periods = 5.2 + 7.9 mmHg; $p < .02$), and a similar pattern was observed for SBP (M difference = 8.4 + 13.9 mmHg; $p < .07$). In contrast, no significant differences were observed in BP responses across these two time periods in wives ($p > .70$). (Neither group of women evidenced differences in HR responses.)

Because daughters, relative to wives, showed significant between-group as well as within-group differences in ambulatory hemodynamic responses when the care recipient was present as opposed to absent, additional within-group analyses (paired-comparison *t* tests) were employed to explore differences in other psychosocial variables during these two time periods within the daughter group. The results of these exploratory analyses are shown in Table 3.

TABLE 3
For Daughters, Mean Ratings (± Standard Deviation) on Affective and Cognitive Variables Assessed in the Natural Setting During the Period of the Day When the Care Recipient Was Either Present or Absent ($n = 36$)

Variable[a]	Care Recipient Absent	Care Recipient Absent
Mental workload[b]	1.6 ± 0.5	1.2 ± 0.3
Emotional upset[c]	2.6 ± 1.4	1.5 ± 0.7
Anger[b]	2.1 ± 1.0	1.3 ± 0.5
Tension or anxiety[b]	2.9 ± 1.2	1.8 ± 1.0
Sadness[d]	1.9 ± 1.7	1.4 ± 0.8
Sleepiness	2.2 ± 1.9	2.9 ± 1.9
Happiness	5.0 ± 2.4	4.9 ± 2.1
Level of demands[c]	4.0 ± 1.5	2.6 ± 1.5
Demands relative to usual[c]	1.9 ± 0.5	1.5 ± 0.4
Feelings of control over situation[c]	6.5 ± 2.3	7.4 ± 2.0

[a]Rated on a 10-point Likert scale ranging from 1 (*low*) to 10 (*high*). [b]Time periods different at $p < .002$. [c]Time periods different at $p < .0006$. [d]Time periods different at $p < .05$. [e]Time periods different at $p < .02$.

Of the 10 affective and cognitive variables assessed via the portable computerized diary, daughters reported significantly more negative levels on 8 of the variables when the care recipient was present as opposed to absent ($p < .04$). The only 2 variables for which such differences were not reported were sleepiness and happiness. In contrast, wives reported significantly more negative levels on only 2 of the 10 affective and cognitive variables when the care recipient was present as opposed to absent (level of demands and level of demands compared to usual; $p < .03$).

Although daughter caregivers rated their affective and cognitive states significantly more negatively when the care recipient was present, the overall mean ratings for these variables, similar to those for wives, were not high, suggesting that in general they were coping adequately with their situation.

DISCUSSION

This study represents the second systematic investigation of hemodynamic responses in the natural environment among older female caregivers. The results of this study corroborate the findings from the original investigation by suggesting that increased hemodynamic responses accompany that portion of the day when daughter caregivers are in the presence of their care recipient (King et al., 1994). The findings of this study also extend the original study results by indicating that increased hemodynamic responses may occur only in daughter, as opposed to wife, caregivers. As reflected in the diary data, these differences were not due to differences in posture, physical activity, or other behavioral factors (e.g., caffeine, tobacco, medication intake) occurring throughout the day. In contrast to the wife-daughter differences found in the natural setting, no between-group differences in hemodynamic response were found in the two standard laboratory-based challenges. This suggests that the greater physiological responsiveness on the part of daughters in the natural setting was not due simply to a general predisposition toward higher levels of physiological responsiveness in that group. The assumption that laboratory-based cardiovascular reactivity procedures capture important dispositional tendencies that carry over into more natural settings has been shown to be valid in some situations (Abel & Larkin, 1991; Matthews, Owens, Allen, & Stoney, 1992). However, this is the first study to evaluate the relation between laboratory-based hemodynamic responses and responses occurring in the natural setting in a caregiving sample—a sample for whom, by virtue of its chronic stress levels and increased morbidity and mortality risk, such questions take on particular importance. Our results suggest that laboratory measurement may not adequately capture differences in hemodynamic functioning observed in the natural environment for at least some caregiver samples.

In light of growing evidence indicating an increased probability of morbidity and mortality outcomes accompanying chronic caregiving duties, an increased focus on potential physiological, behavioral, and psychosocial pathways serving as potential mediators of those relations has been recommended (Schulz & Beach, 1999; Vitaliano et al., 1994). This investigation suggests acute hemodynamic variability in the presence of the care recipient as one possible pathway for some groups of caregivers (notably, daughters) that merits further study. Although the mean ambulatory BP levels across the day for daughters and wives generally remained in the normotensive range, frequent increases in BP throughout the day in response to psychosocial stress may, at least in some individuals, contribute to target organ damage, such as left ventricular hypertrophy, which has been found to be an independent predictor of cardiovascular morbidity (Casale et al., 1986; Pickering et al., 1991). In addition, the increases in BP and HR among daughters in the presence of the care recipient provide physiological evidence in support of the distressing social interactions reported by daughters when the care recipient was present as opposed to absent. The greater frequency of stressful interactions among daughters relative to wives underscores the potential role conflicts that may be more common in many child, relative to spousal, caregiving situations (Skaff & Pearlin, 1992; Strawbridge et al., 1997; Young & Kahana, 1989). It was notable that although the majority of these stressful interactions occurred with the care recipient, another important source of negative interactions for daughter caregivers was other family members. Studies by Russo and Vitaliano (1995), as well as others (Pearlin, Mullan, Semple, & Skaff, 1990; Schuster, Kessler, & Aseltine, 1990), have underscored the potentially iatrogenic effects of interpersonal conflicts with family members in addition to the care recipient on caregiver burden and distress. Other studies of caregivers have indicated that positive forms of social participation and emotional support may be especially important in mitigating depressive symptoms in daughters relative to wives (Li, Seltzer, & Greenberg, 1997). Our results suggest that such forms of positive social and emotional support might also be indicated to help buttress daughters against the greater frequency of negative interpersonal interactions that they may experience with a variety of family members in the presence of the care recipient. In addition, interventions that specifically teach methods of appropriate conflict resolution for caregivers and their families may provide a means for diminishing caregiver stress and physiological responsivity.

As part of this investigation, we conducted a series of analyses to evaluate the potential effects on hemodynamic response of the several demographic variables that differed between wives and daughters (e.g., age, employment status, marital status, care recipient gender, number of people living in the household). Although, given the study design, we cannot fully rule out the potential effects of such variables on the outcomes of interest, the lack of significant effects found for such variables makes it less likely that they were substantially responsible for the results. It should be noted that all of these demographic variables reflect natural differences implicit in being a caregiving daughter versus wife (National Alliance for Caregiving and the American Association of Retired Persons, 1997). That is, across the caregiving population as a whole, daughters tend to be younger than wives, by extension more of them are employed relative to wives, and they tend to have a greater number of people living in their households (due to the presence, often, of their spouse and children; National Alliance for Caregiving and the American Association of Retired Persons, 1997). They therefore often face a potentially greater level of role conflict given the greater number of social roles that they typically face (Skaff & Pearlin, 1992; Strawbridge et al., 1997).

Given the relatively small number of participants being evaluated, caution must be applied with respect to the strength and generalizability of the conclusions that can be drawn. Additional research is required to evaluate the generalizability of our results to different populations of caregivers, including persons of different ethnicity, gender, age, familial relationship (e.g., daughters-in-law), and differing caregiving situations. For example, this sample of daughter and wife caregivers was living with their care recipient. Other studies of daughter caregivers have included only daughters *not* living with their care recipient (Stephens & Townsend, 1997), or a mix of daughters living with or independent of the impaired parent (Martire, Stephens, & Atienza, 1997). Similarly, caregivers in this study were caring for relatives with dementia, as opposed to those with physical health impairments only or a mixed sample of care recipients. In light of the fact that daughters had, on average, a greater number of people living in their households relative to wives, it would also be useful, as noted earlier, to better understand how these additional household relationships could influence caregiver stress. This is particularly true in light of the frequency with which daughter caregivers reported distressing interactions with other family members.

Our results support other investigations indicating the potentially detrimental impact, in both psychosocial and physical arenas, on women serving as family caregivers for an older relative. In addition, the results add to the small body of research indicating that the specific set of circumstances that often accompany home caregiving may have negative acute effects on both psychosocial and physiological responses, especially in daughters. In particular, developing interventions aimed at diminishing the effects of negative interactions on acute physiological as well as emotional responses to stress may benefit the caregiver as well as her family.

REFERENCES

Abel, J. L., & Larkin, K. T. (1991). Assessment of cardiovascular reactivity across laboratory and natural settings. *Journal of Psychosomatic Research, 35,* 365–373.

Alspaugh, M. E. L., Stephens, M. A. P., Townsend, A. L., Zarit, S. H., & Greene, R. (1999). Longitudinal patterns of risk for depression in dementia caregivers: Objective and subjective primary stress as predictors. *Psychology and Aging, 14,* 34–43.

American College of Sports Medicine. (1986). *Guidelines for exercise testing and prescription* (3rd ed.). Philadelphia: Lea & Febiger.

Carels, R. A., Szczepanski, R., Blumenthal, J. A., & Sherwood, A. (1998). Blood pressure reactivity and marital distress in employed women. *Psychosomatic Medicine, 60,* 639–643.

Casale, P. N., Devereux, R. B., Milner, M., Zullo, G., Harshfield, G. A., Pickering, T. G., & Laragh, J. H. (1986). Value of echocardiographic measurement of left ventricular mass in predicting cardiovascular morbid events in hypertensive men. *Annals of Internal Medicine, 105,* 173–178.

Christensen, K. A., Stephens, M. A. P., & Townsend, A. L. (1998). Mastery in women's multiple roles and well-being: Adult daughters providing care to impaired parents. *Health Psychology, 17,* 163–171.

Ewart, C. K., & Koldner, K. B. (1991). Predicting ambulatory blood pressure during school: Effectiveness of social and nonsocial reactive tasks in Black and White adolescents. *Psychophysiology, 26,* 30–38.

Goode, K. T., Haley, W. E., Roth, D. L., & Ford, G. R. (1998). Predicting longitudinal changes in caregiver physical and mental health: A stress process model. *Health Psychology, 17,* 190–198.

Kiecolt-Glaser, J. K., Marucha, P. T., Malarkey, W. B., Mercado, A.M., & Glaser, R. (1995). Slowing of wound healing by psychological stress. *Lancet, 346,* 1194–1196.

King, A. C., & Brassington, G. (1997). Enhancing physical and psychological functioning in older family caregivers: The role of regular physical activity. *Annals of Behavioral Medicine, 19,* 91–100.

King, A. C., Oka, R. K., & Young, D. R. (1994). Ambulatory blood pressure and heart rate responses to the stress of work and caregiving in older women. *Journal of Gerontology: Medical Sciences, 49,* M239–M245.

King, A. C., Pruitt, L. A., Phillips, W., Oka, R., Rodenburg, A., & Haskell, W. L. (2000). Comparative effects of two physical activity programs on measured and perceived physical functioning and other health-related quality of life outcomes in older adults. *Journal of Gerontology: Medical Sciences, 55A,* M74–M83.

King, A. C., Taylor, C. B., Albright, C. A., & Haskell, W. L. (1990). The relationship between repressive and defensive coping styles and blood pressure responses in healthy, middle-aged men and women. *Journal of Psychosomatic Research, 34,* 461–471.

Kral, B. G., Becker, L. C., Blumenthal, R. S., Aversano, T., Fleisher, L. A., Yook, R. M., & Becker, D. M. (1997). Exaggerated reactivity to mental stress is associated with exercise-induced myocardial ischemia in an asymptomatic high-risk population. *Circulation, 96,* 4246–4253.

Lee, C., & Porteous, J. (1998). Family caregiving in the lives of middle-aged Australian women: Health, stress, and adjustment. *Annals of Behavioral Medicine, 20*(Suppl. S170).

Li, L. W., Seltzer, M. M., & Greenberg, J. S. (1997). Social support and depressive symptoms: Differential patterns in wife and daughter caregivers. *Journal of Gerontology: Social Sciences, 52B,* S200–S211.

Martire, L. M., Stephens, M. A. P., & Atienza, A. A. (1997). The interplay of work and caregiving: Relationships between role satisfactions, role involvement, and caregivers' well- being. *Journal of Gerontology: Social Sciences, 52B,* S279–S289.

Matthews, K. A., Owens, J. F., Allen, M. T., & Stoney, C. M. (1992). Do cardiovascular responses to laboratory stress relate to ambulatory blood pressure levels? Yes, in some of the people, some of the time. *Psychosomatic Medicine, 54,* 686–697.

Matthews, K. A., Weiss, S. M., Detre, T., Dembroski, T. M., Falkner, B., Manuck, S. B., & Williams, J., R. B. (Eds.). (1986). *Handbook of stress, reactivity, and cardiovascular disease.* New York: Wiley.

Mills, P. J., Yi, H., Ziegler, M., Patterson, T., & Grant, I. (1999). Vulnerable caregivers of patients with Alzheimer's disease have a deficit in circulating CD62L–T lymphocytes. *Psychosomatic Medicine, 61,* 168–174.

National Alliance for Caregiving and the American Association of Retired Persons. (1997). *Family caregiving in the U.S.: Findings from a national survey* . Bethesda, MD: Author.

Ory, M. G., Hofffman, R. R. I., Yee, J. L., Tennstedt, S., & Schulz, R. (1999). Prevalence and impact of caregiving: A detailed comparison between dementia and nondementia caregivers. *The Gerontologist, 39,* 177–185.

Pearlin, L., Mullan, J. T., Semple, S. J., & Skaff, M. M. (1990). Caregiving and the stress process: An overview of concepts and their measures. *The Gerontologist, 30,* 583–594.

Pickering, T. G., James, G. D., Schnall, P. L., Schlussel, Y. R., Pieper, C. F., Gerin, W., & Karasek, R. A. (1991). Occupational stress and blood pressure: Studies in working men and women. In M. Frankenhaeuser, U. Lundberg, & M. Chesney (Eds.), *Women, work, and health: Stress and opportunities* (pp. 171–186). New York: Plenum.

Russo, J., & Vitaliano, P. P. (1995). Life events as correlates of burden in spouse caregivers of persons with Alzheimer's disease. *Experimental Aging Research, 21,* 273–294.

Russo, J., Vitaliano, P. P., Brewer, D. D., Katon, W., & Becker, J. (1995). Psychiatric disorders in spouse caregivers of care recipients with Alzheimer's disease and matched controls: A diathesis-stress model of psychopathology. *Journal of Abnormal Psychology, 104,* 197–204.

Schulz, R., & Beach, S. R. (1999). Caregiving as a risk factor for mortality: The Caregiver Health Effects study. *Journal of the American Medical Association, 282,* 2215–2219.

Schulz, R., O'Brien, A. T., Bookwala, M. S., & Fleissner, K. (1995). Psychiatric and physical morbidity effects of dementia caregiving: Prevalence, correlates, and causes. *The Gerontologist, 35,* 771–791.

Schuster, T. L., Kessler, R. C., & Aseltine, R. H. (1990). Supportive interactions, negative interactions, and depressed mood. *American Journal of Community Psychology, 18,* 423–438.

Skaff, M. M., & Pearlin, L. I. (1992). Caregiving: Role engulfment and the loss of self. *The Gerontologist, 32,* 656–664.

Stephens, M. A. P., & Townsend, A. L. (1997). Stress of parent care: Positive and negative effects of women's other roles. *Psychology and Aging, 12,* 376–386.

Stone, R., Cafferata, G. L., & Sangl, J. (1987). Caregivers of the frail elderly: A national profile. *The Gerontologist, 27,* 616–626.

Strawbridge, W. J., Wallhagen, M. I., Shemea, S. J., & Kaplan, G. A. (1997). New burdens or more of the same? Comparing grandparent, spouse, and adult–child caregivers. *The Gerontologist, 37,* 505–510.

Taylor, C. B., Fried, L., & Kenardy, J. (1990). The use of a real-time computer diary for data acquisition and processing. *Behavior Research and Therapy, 21,* 93–97.

Vitaliano, P. P., Dougherty, C. M., & Siegler, I. C. (1994). Biopsychosocial risks for cardiovascular disease in spouse caregivers of persons with Alzheimer's disease. In R. P. Abeles, H. C. Gift, & M. G. Ory (Eds.), *Aging and quality of life* (pp. 145–159). New York: Springer.

Vitaliano, P. P., Russo, J., Bailey, S. L., Young, H. M., & McCann, B. S. (1993). Psychosocial factors associated with cardiovascular reactivity in older adults. *Psychosomatic Medicine, 55,* 164–177.

Vitaliano, P. P., Russo, J., Young, H. M., Becker, J., & Maiuro, R. D. (1991). The screen for caregiver burden. *The Gerontologist, 31,* 76–83.

Vitaliano, P. P., Russo, J., Young, H. M., Teri, L., & Maiuro, R. D. (1991). Predictors of burden in spouse caregivers of individuals with Alzheimer's disease. *Psychology and Aging, 6,* 392–402.

Vitaliano, P. P., Scanlan, J. M., Siegler, I. C., McCormick, W. C., & Knopp, R. H. (1998). Coronary heart disease moderates the relationship of chronic stress with the metabolic syndrome. *Health Psychology, 17,* 520–529.

White, W. B., Lund-Johansen, P., & McCabe, E. J. (1989). Clinical evaluation of the Colin ABPM 630 at rest and during exercise: An ambulatory blood pressure monitor with gas-powered cuff inflation. *Journal of Hypertension, 7,* 477–483.

White, W. B., Lund-Johansen, P., & Omvik, P. (1990). Assessment of four ambulatory blood pressure monitors and measurements of clinicians versus intra-arterial blood pressure at rest and during exercise. *American Journal of Cardiology, 65,* 60–66.

Wilcox, S., & King, A. C. (1999). Sleep complaints in older women who are family caregivers. *Journal of Gerontology: Psychological Sciences, 54B,* P189–P198.

Wu, H., Wang, J., Cacioppo, J. T., Glaser, R., Kiecolt-Glaser, J. K., & Malarkey, W. B. (1999). Chronic stress associated with spousal caregiving of patients with Alzheimer's dementia is associated with downregulation of B-lymphocyte GH mRNA. *Journal of Gerontology: Medical Sciences, 54A,* M212–M215.

Young, R. F., & Kahana, E. (1989). Specifying caregiver outcomes: Gender and relationship aspects of caregiving strain. *The Gerontologist, 29,* 660–666.

INTERNATIONAL JOURNAL OF BEHAVIORAL MEDICINE, 9(3), 195–215

Number of Social Roles, Health, and Well-Being in Three Generations of Australian Women

Christina Lee and Jennifer R. Powers

The relation between multiple social roles and health is a particular issue for women, who continue to take major responsibility for childcare and domestic labor despite increasing levels of involvement in the paid workforce. This article analyzes Survey 1 data from the Australian Longitudinal Survey on Women's Health to explore relations between role occupancy and health, well-being, and health service use in three generations of Australian women. A total of 41,818 women in three age groups (young, 18–23; mid-age, 40–45; older, 70–75) responded to mailed surveys. Young and mid-age women were classified according to their occupancy of five roles—paid worker, partner, mother, student, and family caregiver—whereas older women were classified according to occupancy of partner and caregiver roles only. Common symptoms (headaches, tiredness, back pain, difficulty sleeping), diagnosis of chronic illness, and use of health services were compared across groups characterized by number of roles. Comparisons were also conducted on the physical and mental component scores of the SF–36 and perceived stress, with and without adjustment for confounders. Among young women, the best health was associated with occupancy of one role; among mid-age women, those with three or more roles were in the best health; and for older women, those with one role were in the best health. Young women with none or with four or more roles, and mid-age and older women with none of the defined social roles tended to be in the poorest health. Different patterns of results may be explained by differences in the extent to which women at different life stages feel committed to various social roles, and to the extent to which they are able to draw on social, material, and economic supports.

Christina Lee and Jennifer R. Powers, Research Centre for Gender and Health, University of Newcastle, Callaghan, Australia.

The Australian Longitudinal Study on Women's Health, of which this research is a part, is funded by the Australian Commonwealth Department of Health and Aged Care.

Correspondence concerning this article should be addressed to Christina Lee, Director, Research Centre for Gender and Health, University of Newcastle, Callaghan, NSW 2308 Australia. E-mail: whcel@mail.newcastle.edu.au

Key words: physical health, SF - 36, social roles, stress, symptoms, women

Understanding the nature of the relation between social roles and health is relevant to the development of health policy and the provision of appropriate health services throughout the lifespan. This is particularly the case for women in the current social context (Spurlock, 1995). Although women's expectations concerning employment and equality have changed radically in the past few decades, at the same time women continue to take major responsibility for childcare and unpaid domestic labor (e.g., Bittman, 1992). Holding multiple social roles has an impact on women's health and well-being, and at a broader level on the development of social policy that promotes healthy women, healthy families, and healthy communities (Aube, Fleury, & Smetana, 2000).

This article focuses on the extent to which the number of social roles that a woman occupies (as distinct from the specific types of roles she has) is associated with a range of measures of health. There exist several models of the relations between a woman's number of simultaneous social roles and her well-being (Stephens & Franks, 1999). The *scarcity hypothesis* holds that occupancy of more than one social role (e.g., paid worker and parent) will cause stress and ill-health to the extent that the demands of those roles interfere with each other (role conflict) or create an excessive overall workload (role overload). This model is supported by at least some evidence that combinations of roles can result in high levels of guilt and anxiety (e.g., Baruch & Barnett, 1986) and have a negative effect on women's physical health (e.g., Lundberg, 1996).

By contrast, the *enhancement hypothesis* holds that occupying several social roles provides the individual with a range of sources of positive social interaction, pleasurable activity, achievement, and status, and thus benefits well-being.

It is certainly not the case that more roles automatically means more stress. For example, Forgays and Forgays (1993) found that women who combined paid work, marriage, and motherhood were actually less stressed than married mothers without paid employment. Multiple role occupancy provides both stress and satisfaction in women's lives; several researchers have shown that women with multiple roles report both more strain and more satisfaction than those occupying only one (e.g., Gerson, 1985; Park & Liao, 2000). Thus, occupancy of multiple roles can be simultaneously positive and negative; its effects are influenced by a variety of factors, including psychological characteristics (Moen, Robison, & Dempster-McClain, 1995), the woman's sense that each role is central to her view of herself (Martire, Stephens, & Townsend, 2000), the perceived quality of each role (e.g., Roxburgh, 1997), and her economic ability to outsource some labor and avoid overload (e.g., Wallace, 1999).

It is also possible that different combinations of roles may differ in the extent to which they provide stresses and satisfactions; being a parent and a partner may, for example, be a quite different experience from being a worker and a caregiver. However, this article focuses on the number of simultaneous roles, and leaves the issue of what these specific roles are for a later analysis. The article examines the occupancy of up to five simultaneous roles in the lives of young and mid-age Australian women (worker, partner, mother, caregiver, and student) and of up to two roles in the lives of older women (partner and caregiver). Most literature to date has considered each of these roles in isolation, and we briefly review evidence that suggests each specific role can be characterized by both positive and negative effects on health and well-being.

WORKER

Psychological research has generally accepted uncritically the assumption that paid work will necessarily be problematic for women and not for men; it assumes that, for women, paid work must be added to their "natural" roles as unpaid domestic workers and parents. Women who occupy all three of these roles certainly report strain and conflict (e.g., Spurlock, 1995), but paid work, although stressful, is simultaneously beneficial to women's physical and emotional health. Several longitudinal studies (e.g., Bromberger & Matthews, 1994; Hibbard & Pope, 1991; Waldron, Weiss, & Hughes, 1998; Weatherall, Joshi, & Macran, 1994) have demonstrated that moving into the paid workforce confers a health advantage.

PARTNER

Being married or in a permanent relationship is viewed as both normal and desirable. Australian survey data (Lee, 2001c; Wicks & Mishra, 1998) show that 96% of young women aspire to be married or in a stable relationship by the age of 35; this compares with 81% of mid-age women and 55% of older women who are in permanent relationships (a further 35% of the older women are widows). There is strong epidemiological evidence that married women have lower all-cause mortality and better physical health than the unmarried (e.g., Cheung, 2000; Johnson, Backlund, Sorlie, & Loveless, 2000). Longitudinal research (e.g., Waldron, Hughes, & Brooks, 1996) indicates that, for women in particular, this effect can be explained both by selection—healthy women are more likely to marry and to remain married—and protection—marriage tends to improve women's health. These effects, however, are found only among the dwindling minority of women who do not have paid work, suggesting that marriage and paid work provide similar benefits and can to some extent substitute for each other (Waldron et al., 1998).

PARENT

Caring for children is stressful but, especially for those women who find the role enjoyable and rewarding, provides benefits that may improve women's ability to cope with stress and strain from the occupancy of other roles. For example, Barnett, Marshall, and Singer (1992) found that reductions in job quality led to increased distress among single women, but not among those with husbands and children. Increased job pressure seemed to be buffered by sources of satisfaction in the women's other roles. Most women want children, and most do become mothers. In Australia, 92% of young women want at least one child by the age of 35 (Wicks & Mishra, 1998), whereas 91% of mid-age and older women have at least one child in their lifetime (Brown, Young, & Byles, 1999; Lee, 2001c). Despite the high social and personal value placed on motherhood, women who combine motherhood and paid work roles do report high levels of role strain (e.g., Reifman, Biernat, & Lang, 1991). On the other hand, longitudinal survey research from the United States (Waldron et al., 1998) and the United Kingdom (Weatherall et al., 1994) has found no evidence that the combination of motherhood and paid employment had any negative effect on physical health.

STUDENT

The impact of the student role and its combination with other social roles has received relatively little attention, perhaps because of an assumption that students do not generally have other roles. In Australia in 2000, however, 43% of all university students were aged over 30 and 41% were studying on a part-time or external basis (Department of Education, Training & Youth Affairs, 2001), suggesting that a high proportion of people occupying a student role will be combining this with paid work, parenthood, and other demanding social roles. Examining the lives of women combining study with paid work and family responsibilities, Home (1997, 1998) identified significant levels of role strain and stress. Gerson (1985) found that women with children who were also studying reported both more strain and more gratification than unemployed, nonstudying mothers. Neither study, however, examined physical or emotional health.

CAREGIVER

Increasing interest in the stresses associated with family caregiving (e.g., Lee, 1999) has led to research that assesses the impact of this role on women's perceived stress, their physical and emotional health, and their sense of role strain and conflict (Doress-Worters, 1994; Voydanoff & Donnelly, 1999). A recent review of the evidence (Lee, 1999) concluded that caregiving was associated with role strain and poor emotional health, but that there was little evidence for any effect on physical health. As with other roles, the nature of the caregiving role and the extent of social supports and satisfactions will mediate the relation between role occupancy and health. Stephens, Townsend, Martire, and Druley (2001), for example, found that women who cared for ill or frail parents at home in addition to being mothers, wives, and paid workers generally experienced at least some role strain, but that strain was mediated by factors such as the degree of the parent's impairment, the age of their children, and their economic status. Caregiving may have different effects at different life stages. Analysis of data from the Women's Health Australia project (Lee, 2001a, 2001b; Lee & Porteous, 2002) has shown a greater health difference between caregivers and noncaregivers in middle age than in old age, but this may result from selection into caregiving roles rather than from the effects of caregiving on health.

NUMBER OF ROLES

The occupancy of any one of the five roles under discussion has been shown to be associated with stress and with gratification. The final effect on any individual is likely to depend on the total number of roles as well as on the individual's ability to cope with that role. Ability to cope, in turn, will be mediated both by physical health and by sociodemographic factors. This article uses data from the Australian Longitudinal Survey on Women's Health (Women's Health Australia) to examine up to five different social roles in the lives of three age cohorts of Australian women. It examines the relation between the number of roles occupied by these women and their physical health, symptoms, emotional well-being, and health service use, separately in three different age cohorts. Cross-sectional relations between health and role occupancy may be explained by the effects of multiple roles on health, by the effects of health on ability to occupy multiple roles, or by the effects of confounders on both sets of variables. Thus, analysis is conducted both with and without adjustment for possible health-related and sociodemographic confounders.

METHOD

Background

Women's Health Australia, a longitudinal survey of the health and well-being of three cohorts of Australian women, has been described in detail elsewhere (Brown et al., 1998; Lee, 2001c). The main project involves mailed surveys to collect self-report data on health and related variables from three cohorts of Australian women, who were aged 18 to 23 years ("young"), 45 to 50 years ("mid-age"), and 70 to 75 years ("older") when the project began in 1996. Over 40,000 women were recruited on a random basis from the Australian population, with the comprehensive national health insurance database (Medicare) as the sampling frame and systematic over-representation of women living in rural and remote areas. This database encompasses all permanent residents of Australia, including migrants and refugees.

The project is designed to run for 20 years, so that the "young" cohort can be tracked through early and middle adulthood; the "mid-age" cohort through menopause, later middle age, and early old age; and the "older" cohort through their 70s, 80s, and beyond. The aim is to conduct a series of interlocking data analyses to develop an understanding of structural and societal factors that affect the health and well-being of women to inform government health policy in the 21st century (Lee, 2001c).

Participants

This analysis focuses on Survey 1 data for all three cohorts. A total of 14,779 young women, 14,100 mid-age women, and 12,939 older women responded to Survey 1 in 1996 (an overall response rate of 40%). Social role data were available for 41,175 women (98%) who were included in this analysis. Comparisons with census data from the Australian Bureau of Statistics indicate that the samples were demographically representative of Australian women in these age groups, with a slight over-representation of married, Australian-born, and highly educated subgroups (Brown et al., 1998).

Survey

Respondents completed a 24-page survey comprising over 300 items that addressed health status, health service use and satisfaction, health-related behaviors, and sociodemographic variables. The surveys for the three age groups differed slightly so that women were not asked age-inappropriate questions. This analysis used the following variables.

Social roles.   Presence or absence of each of five social roles was defined as follows. *Worker:* women who were in paid employment on a full- or part-time basis, or worked on an unpaid basis in a family business, scored 1; all others scored 0. *Partner:* women who reported currently living in a marriage or de facto relationship scored 1; all others scored 0. *Parent:* women who reported having children living with them, regardless of whether these were their own or someone else's children, scored 1; all others scored 0. *Student:* those currently studying full-time or part-time scored 1; all others scored 0. *Caregiver:* those who reported that they "provided care on a regular basis to another person because of their long-term illness, frailty or disability" scored 1; all others scored 0.

Data on all five possible roles were used for women in the young and mid-age cohorts; for the older cohort (aged 70–75), data on partner and care-giver roles only were used. Although approximately 1% of older women did live with their adult children and grandchildren, it was not clear that they took a parenting role. Numbers who were in paid work or studying were too small for statistical analysis.

Sociodemographic variables are described in Table 1.

Health and well-being.   The Medical Outcomes Study Short Form (SF–36, Ware & Sherbourne, 1992), a comprehensive measure of health-related quality of life, was used to measure perceived general health and well-being. Summary physical component scores (PCS) and mental component scores (MCS) were derived and standardized so that a score below 50 indicates worse, and greater than 50 indicates better, health than the population mean (Mishra & Schofield, 1998).

TABLE 1
Weighted Percentages for Sociodemographic Characteristics of the Three Age Cohorts

	Young[a]	Mid[b]	Old[c]
Country of birth			
Australia	89.6	70.1	73.1
Elsewhere	10.4	29.9	26.9
Marital status			
Married/defacto	20.3	80.8	55.4
Divorced/separated	0.8	13.2	6.3
Never married	78.8	3.9	3.2
Widowed	0.1	2.1	35.1
Highest qualifications			
Some schooling	14.6	46.2	71.0
Finished high school	55.3	17.4	13.2
Further education	30.1	36.3	15.9
How do you manage on the income you have available?			
Easy	13.2	16.0	22.3
Not too bad	36.0	41.9	50.9
Difficult some of the time	32.8	27.6	19.6
Difficult all the time/impossible	18.0	14.4	7.2

Percentages weighted to account for over-sampling of rural and remote women.
Numbers vary due to small percentages of missing data.
[a]$n = 14,632$. [b]$n = 13,869$. [c]$n = 12,674$.

1. Chronic illness: Each survey included a list of major diagnoses and women indicated whether they had been diagnosed with each. For the young women, this included diabetes, heart disease, hypertension, asthma, and cancer; the surveys for the mid-age and older women included these as well as stroke, thrombosis, bronchitis/emphysema, and osteoporosis. For the purposes of analysis, women who indicated that they had ever been diagnosed with three or more of the listed conditions were defined as "chronically ill."

2. Symptoms: Each survey included a list of common symptoms, and women were asked to rate whether they had experienced each symptom often, sometimes, rarely, or never in the previous 12 months. The list of symptoms differed between age groups, but this analysis used four items that were included in all three groups: headaches, tiredness, back pain, and difficulty sleeping. For analysis, respondents were dichotomized into those reporting each symptom *often* and those reporting it *sometimes, rarely,* or *never.*

3. Stress: A series of items asked women to rate the extent to which they were stressed by a range of aspects of their lives, including their own health, the health of family members, living arrangements, money, and relationships. The young and mid-age women were also asked about work and study. The mean response to these items was used as a measure of stress, with a theoretical range from 0, indicating *no stress,* to 4, indicating *extreme stress* (Bell & Lee, in press).

4. Health service use: Three variables were used to assess level of health service use. Respondents specified the number of general medical practitioner visits and medical specialist visits and whether they had been admitted to the hospital in the previous year. Those who reported seven or more general medical practitioner visits, seven or more specialist visits, or any hospital admission were categorized as *high* health service users on that variable.

Smoking: Current smoking status was dichotomized as smoker or nonsmoker.

Statistical Analyses

All analyses were performed taking the over-sampling in rural and remote areas into account. Differences in proportions were examined using chi-square tests. The distributions of mean stress, PCS, and MCS were checked for normality, and the least squares mean option in the general linear model procedure was used to estimate means and 95% confidence intervals. Analysis was conducted both with and without adjustment for the potential confounders of country of birth, qualifications, ability to manage on available income, smoking, and number of chronic illnesses (0, 1, 2, 3, or more).

With large sample sizes, small differences in means may be statistically significant but not clinically significant. Although no definitive guidelines for clinical significance of PCS and MCS exist, normative data from the 1995 Australian National Health Survey (Australian Bureau of Statistics, 1997) show that the presence of one serious physical condition such as cancer, diabetes, hypertension, or arthritis is associated with a reduction of three points in PCS and two points in MCS.

Analyses were conducted both with and without participants who reported being pregnant at the time of data collection (young: $n = 438, 3\%$; mid-age: $n = 103, 0.7\%$). Results were essentially the same, so the full data sets only are reported.

RESULTS

Table 1 provides sociodemographic data for each of the three age cohorts in this analysis, whereas Table 2 shows the percentage of women in each age group who occupy each of five specified roles and the percentage holding each number of roles.

TABLE 2
Social Roles (%) for Three Age Cohorts

Social Role	Young (n = 14,632)		Mid (n = 13,869)		Old (n = 12,674)	
Worker[a]	52.4		74.6			
Partner	20.3		80.8		55.2	
Parent[a]	7.5		64.4			
Student[a]	49.3		8.7			
Caregiver	7.7		20.1		17.1	
Number of Roles	n	%	n	%	n	%
0	766	5.2	212	1.5	4863	38.4
1	8588	58.7	1675	12.1	6447	50.9
2	4439	30.3	4797	34.6	1364	10.8
3	774	5.3	5606	40.4		
4	63	0.4	1476	10.6		
5	2	0	103	0.8		

Note. Percentages weighted to account for over-sampling of rural and remote women.
[a]Young and mid-age women only.

TABLE 3
Percentage of Women in Three Age Cohorts at Each Level of a Variety
of Health Indicators by Number of Social Roles

	Young		Mid		Old	
Number of Social Roles	%	χ^2	%	χ^2	%	χ^2
Often had headaches/migraine in the last 12 months						
0	20.3		21.5			6.9
1	17.5		18.2			7.0
2	18.5	39.4***	18.3	5.8	8.3	3.1
3	25.5		16.9			
4 or 5	33.5		17.5			
Often had constant tiredness in the last 12 months						
0	16.3		40.2		13.6	
1	17.4		20.0		11.7	
2	19.7	45.0***	18.9	66.2***	13.4	10.1**
3	25.6		18.1			
4 or 5	31.7		19.0			
Often had back pain in the last 12 months						
0	12.6		38.3		25.5	
1	10.7		24.5		21.8	
2	13.4	43.3***	20.3	80.1***	24.8	21.2***
3	17.3		18.2			
4 or 5	13.8		18.0			
Often had difficulty sleeping in the last 12 months						
0	17.3		33.6		17.1	
1	9.3		20.6		15.3	
2	9.4	51.6***	17.2	94.2***	16.8	7.2*
3	10.8		14.1			
4 or 5	13.3		15.0			
Ever diagnosed with three or more chronic conditions						
0	0.4		20.0		21.2	
1	0.2		7.4		17.4	
2	0.3	67.2***	5.7	178.6***	15.7	47.2***
3	0.7		4.5			
4 or 5	0	4.9				
Seven or more visits to a general medical practitioner in last 12 months						
0	20.4		45.7		35.1	
1	14.2		23.4		30.7	
2	18.5	193.5***	15.7	354.8***	25.8	56.4***
3	24.3		11.2			
4 or 5	29.5	11.9				

(Continued)

TABLE 3
(Continued)

Number of Social Roles	Young		Mid		Old	
	%	χ^2	%	χ^2	%	χ^2
Seven or more visits to a specialist in the last 12 months						
0	2.3		19.9		5.3	
1	1.6	6.4		4.7		
2	2.6	63.3***	86.7***	4.1	13.7	
		4.52				
3	3.1		2.6			
4 or 5	6.4	1.7				
Admitted to the hospital in the last 12 months						
0	18.6		26.0		25.3	
1	14.3		18.3		22.5	
2	20.5	137.4***	16.3	32.0***	18.7	28.9***
3	26.3		14.5			
4 or 5	30.8		16.4			

Note. Percentages were weighted to account for over-sampling of rural and remote women and roles were collapsed to 3 (*young*) and 4 (*mid*) for analyses.
*$p < .05$. **$p < .01$. ***$p < .0001$.

Young women were most likely to have only one role: These women (59% of the total) were most likely to be students (50%) or workers (43%). Thirty percent of young women had two roles and these were most likely to be worker/student (37%) or worker/partner (28%). The parent role was the least frequently endorsed (7.5%) and the majority of those who had a parent role cared for one child. Most young women with no roles were actively looking for work (71%) and most were living with their parents (58%).

Mid-age women were most likely to endorse three roles (40%), although two roles were also common (35%). The predominant triple role was partner/worker/parent (74%), whereas double roles included partner/worker (44%), partner/parent (28%), and worker/parent (18%). Those who were defined as having a parent role (i.e., had a child at home) were most likely to have a child over the age of 15, although 41% of mid-age parents cared for a younger child.

Older women only had the opportunity to endorse "partner" or "caregiver" roles. The major single role for older women was partner (88%), and by definition all those with two roles were combining partner and caregiver roles, although it is important to note that some were providing care to someone other than their partner.

Tables 3, 4, 5, and 6 show the relation between number of roles and the outcome variables for each age group separately. For the purposes of analysis, young women

TABLE 4
Physical and Mental Health Component Scores (PCS and MCS) and Mean Stress Scores for the Young Cohort (n = 14,622)[a]

Number of Social Roles	(PCS)[b] Unadjusted 95% CI	M	Adjusted 95% CI	M	(MCS)[b] Unadjusted 95% CI	M	Adjusted 95% CI	M	Mean Stress[c] Unadjusted M	95% CI	Adjusted 95% CI	M
0	46.4; 47.8	47.1	42.6; 44.9	43.7	47.8; 49.2	48.5	46.7; 48.9	47.8	0.98	0.94; 1.02	0.93; 1.05	0.97
1	50.5; 50.9	50.7	44.8; 46.5	45.7	50.0; 50.4	50.2	46.9; 48.7		0.91	0.90; 0.93	0.97; 1.07	1.02
2	49.5; 50.1	49.8	44.2; 46.0	45.1	49.8; 50.3	50.1	46.7; 48.5	47.6	0.89	0.87; 0.91	0.96; 1.05	1.01
3 to 5	47.2; 48.6	47.9	42.8; 44.9	43.9	48.3; 49.7	49.0	46.1; 48.2	47.2	0.96	0.92; 1.00	0.99; 1.11	1.05
	$F = 47.3$ $p < .0001$		$F = 15.6$ $p < .0001$		$F = 9.7$ $p < .0001$		$F = 1.1$ $p = .36$		$F = 8.3$ $p < .0001$		$F = 2.7$ $p = .046$	

Note. All means weighted to account for over-sampling in rural and remote areas.
[a]Data are presented both with and without adjustment for country of birth, qualifications, ability to manage on available income, number of chronic illnesses, and smoking status. [b]Higher scores indicate better self-rated health. [c]Higher scores indicate greater stress.

206

TABLE 5

Physical and Mental Health Component Scores (PCS and MCS) and
Mean Stress Scores for the Mid Cohort (N = 13,855)[a]

| Number of Social Role | (PCS)[b] | | | | (MCS)[b] | | | | Mean Stress[c] | | | |
| | Unadjusted | | Adjusted | | Unadjusted | | Adjusted | | Unadjusted | | Adjusted | |
	M	95% CI	M	95% CI	M	95% CI	M	95% CI	M	95% CI	M	95% CI
0	41.1	39.7; 42.4	41.2	39 8; 42.6	42.4	41 0, 43 8	43.2	41.9; 44.6	1.00	0.93; 1.07	0.91	0.85; 0.98
1	48.0	47.5; 48.5	46.2	45.7; 46.7	49.1	48.6; 49.6	48.2	47.7; 48.7	0.73	0.66; 0.69	0.79	0.79; 0.83
2	4.98	49.5; 50 1	47.2	46.9; 47.6	50.3	50.0; 50.6	48.4	48.0; 48.7	0.68	0.66; 0.69	0.81	0.79; 0.83
3	50.9	50.6; 51.2	47.8	47 4; 48.2	50.6	50.4; 50.9	48.4	48.1; 48.8	0.69	0.67; 0.70	0.84	0.82; 0.86
4 to 5	51.3	50.8; 51.8	48.1	47.6; 48 7	50.0	49.5; 50.5	47.7	47.1; 48.2	0.80	0.77; 0.83	0.95	0.92; 0.97
	F = 74.3	p < .0001	F = 28.9	p < .0001	F = 36.8	p < .0001	F = 14.2	p<.0001	F = 36.8	p < .0001	F = 26.3	P < .0001

Note. All means weighted to account for over-sampling in rural and remote areas.

TABLE 6
Physical and Mental Health Component Scores (PCS and MCS)
and Mean Stress Scores for the Old Cohort ($n = 12,672$)[a]

| Number of Social Roles | (PCS)[a] | | | | (MCS)[b] | | | | M Stress[c] | | | |
| | Unadjusted | | Adjusted | | Unadjusted | | Adjusted | | Unadjusted | | Adjusted | |
	M	95% CI	M	95% CI	M	95% CI	M	95% CI	M	95% CI	M	95% CI
0	49.5	49.2; 49.8	49.2	48.7; 49.6	49.7	49.4; 50.0	48.5	48.0; 48.9	0.42	0.40; 0.43	0.51	0.49; 0.53
1	50.3	50.0; 50.5	49.3	48.8; 49.7	50.8	50.6; 51.1	48.9	48.4; 49.4	0.39	0.38; 0.40	0.53	0.51; 0.55
2	50.3	49.7; 50.8	49.1	48.4; 49.7	49.1	48.6; 49.7	47.1	46.4; 47.8	0.56	0.53; 0.58	0.70	0.67; 0.72
	$F = 48.2$	$p < .0001$	$F = 0.3$	$p = .74$	$F = 24.7$	$p < .0001$	$F = 15.7$	$p < .0001$	$F = 76.5$	$p < .0001$	$F = 90.3$	$P < .0001$

Note. All means weighted to account for over-sampling in rural and remote areas.

were categorized into four groups, holding 0, 1, 2, and 3 or more roles; mid-age women were categorized into five groups, holding 0, 1, 2, 3, and 4 or more roles; older women were categorized into three groups, holding 0, 1, and 2 roles, respectively.

Table 3 presents the percentage in each age group who "often" experienced each of four symptoms, were categorized as "chronically ill," and were high users of health services, by number of social roles. The pattern of results, by number of social roles, differed across age groups.

For the four symptoms, the young women with one social role generally had the lowest levels of symptom reporting, whereas those with no social roles and those with multiple roles were more likely to report symptoms. Among the mid-age women, more social roles was associated with lower levels of symptoms reporting; among the older women, one social role (generally "partner") was associated with the lowest level of symptoms. For the three measures of health service use, young women with one social role had the lowest use and those with multiple roles the highest; use increased with increasing number of roles but was also elevated for young women with no social roles. The pattern for mid-age and older women was again different from that for the young women, indicating that those with more roles had lower health service use.

Tables 4, 5, and 6 show mean PCS, MCS, and stress levels for the three cohorts separately. Analysis of variance indicated significant differences across groups defined by number of roles for each variable in each age group, before adjusting for potential confounders. After adjustment, MCS and mean stress were no longer significantly different across groups in the young, nor was PCS in the older cohort. The pattern for young women suggests that those with one social role have the highest level of physical health, whereas those with no or with three or more social roles are in the worst health. For mid-age women, increasing numbers of social roles are consistently associated with better physical health, and one to three roles with the best emotional health and lowest stress. Among older women, physical health does not differ across number of roles, whereas emotional well-being is lowest, and stress highest, among women with two roles.

DISCUSSION

This analysis has examined the relation between multiple role occupancy and a range of measures of physical and emotional well-being in three age cohorts of Australian women. The most striking finding was that the relation between role occupancy and well-being differed across age groups. Among the young women, occupying one social role was associated with the best health. Young women with one social role were predominantly students or in paid work, and these results would appear to support the scarcity hypotheses of role overload or conflict. For these young women, it does seem to be the case that those with no roles and those who occupy three or more roles are generally in worse physical health than those occupying only one. The same pattern of results is found for mental health and for stress, but the effect disappears once the confounders are taken into account, suggesting that the low levels of mental health observed among young women in no or with many roles are explicable by sociodemographic factors and by diagnosed chronic disease.

The results for the mid-age women were entirely different. For these women, more social roles were associated with better physical and emotional health. Generally, mid-age women with three social roles had the healthiest scores on all three outcome variables. Those occupying four or five roles scored better than those with three roles on some variables and worse on others, but their results were somewhat better than those with two roles and definitely better than those who occupied one or no social roles. Mid-age women predominantly combined the three roles of worker, parent, and partner roles, or occupied two of these three. Although these women are almost certain to encounter conflicts in their use of time, these findings support the enhancement hypothesis. Taking confounders into account did not change the pattern of results, suggesting that these differences are not explicable by sociodemographics or by chronic illness.

The design of the surveys meant that older women were only asked about two social roles—partner and caregiver. In this age group, those occupying one role scored best on some outcomes, and those occupying two roles scored best on most of the others. For the older women, occupying either one or two roles was associated with better health than occupying none, but the differences between one and two roles were inconsistent.

Before considering the implications of these findings, it is important to note the cross-sectional nature of this analysis. The relation between number of roles and health is a reciprocal one (Adelmann, Antonucci, Crohan, & Coleman, 1990). Women with poor health may be unable to take on multiple roles, whereas lack of meaningful roles may in turn lead to poor physical and emotional health. For example, a longitudinal survey in New Zealand (Romans, Walton, McNoe, Herbison, & Mullen, 1993) found that women without meaningful work or social roles were those who were most likely to develop psychiatric disorders, but also that those who were experiencing psychological distress and poor health at baseline were most likely to remain without work or family.

Our results show that young women cope best with one role and mid-age women cope best with multiple roles. A number of explanations may be possible. Successful occupancy of multiple roles requires time management skills, self-confidence, and a willingness to deviate from traditional gender expectations (Moen & Yu, 2000), skills that women may acquire as they move through life. The mid-age women occupying multiple roles may have developed these skills over time, suggesting that the younger women may also develop effective coping strategies by the time they reach middle age themselves.

Alternatively, the differing results may arise from differing sociohistorical circumstances. Women who are young adults now have had very different life experiences and expectations from those of their mothers' generation. Young Australian women have very high expectations of their own ability to combine family and career (Wicks & Mishra, 1998). A U.S. survey of mid-age couples, by contrast, showed that the women appeared to have undergone a "scaling-back" process by which high career aspirations were abandoned to accommodate the demands of work and family (Becker & Moen, 1999). It is not clear whether this represents a generational or cultural difference in expectations and attitudes, or whether the young women of today, and their partners, are willing or able to compromise on high expectations to cope with multiple roles as they pass through life.

A third possible explanation of these findings is that the young women occupying multiple roles in this sample are a biased subgroup of women in the 18- to 23-year-old age group. Women who adopt the motherhood role or move into a partnered relationship at this relatively early age are different in many ways from women whose young adult transitions occur "on time" (Brooks-Gunn & Chase-Lansdale, 1995); therefore, they may be less able to cope with multiple role occupancy. As the longitudinal project progresses, it will be possible to examine the extent to which these different hypotheses adequately explain longitudinal trends in the data.

A further, relatively neglected issue that these data identify is that of individuals who have no apparent social roles. In this particular analysis, women with no defined roles represented 5% of the young women, 1.5% of the mid-age women, and 38% of the older women. In general, the young and mid-age women had poor levels of health and well-being. This was particularly notable among the mid-age women, whose SF–36 scores showed clinically significant differences from the other groups, even after adjustment for chronic illness and sociodemographic variables.

Among the young women, those with no roles were most likely to report headaches, sleeping difficulties, and frequent general practitioner visits; to score lowest on the physical and mental components of the SF–36; and to report the highest levels of stress. On the other hand, they had the lowest level of "constant tiredness" and second lowest level of back pain, and were the second lowest users of medical specialists and hospital admissions. This group might include individuals who were physically ill and those who were having difficulties making the normal transitions of late adolescence and early adulthood; the high level of active job-seeking in this group suggests that their lack of defined social roles was the product of circumstance rather than choice. Longitudinally, the project will explore the characteristics of those women who make the important transitions of young adulthood successfully and those who do not.

Among mid-age women, the group with none of the targeted social roles had by far the worst outcomes on every variable assessed. This group included a large proportion of women with multiple chronic illnesses and symptoms, but the effect remained even after adjusting for chronic illness. They were high users of health care services, and even after adjustment their mean scores on the SF–36 physical and mental components were around 5 points lower than other mid-age women, a difference that has been shown to be clinically significant (Australian Bureau of Statistics, 1997).

Although these women had low levels of physical and emotional well-being that could prevent them from occupying social roles, it is also likely that their lack of social roles would serve to maintain their distress. Waldron et al. (1996) found that young and mid-age women who were neither married nor employed had the poorest health and experienced a range of interrelated social and health disadvantages that prevented them from taking on meaningful social roles. Weatherall et al. (1994) found that women with neither paid work nor children at home had the poorest health. Similarly, Dautzenberg, Diederiks, Philipsen, and Tan (1999) found that mid-age women who occupied no social roles had the highest levels of distress, and that those in this situation who took on the usually stressful role of family caregiver actually showed reductions in their distress. Although women occupying no social roles represent a small minority of women in this age group, they are a group who appear particularly vulnerable to poor health.

Among the older sample, those with no social roles scored worst on three of the four symptoms, chronic illness, all measures of health service use, and the physical component score of the SF–36 (although this effect disappeared after adjustment for confounders). Somewhat surprisingly, although, they actually had the lowest levels of headaches and scored better than those with two roles on stress and on the mental component of the SF–36. They represent over a third of the older women, a significantly larger proportion than in the other two age groups, and are less obviously a group in poor health. This is a group who could usefully be investigated in more depth. The question of whether other social roles become increasingly meaningful in later life is worthy of consideration. For example, Moen, Erickson, and Dempster-McClain (2000) showed that retirement home residents considered volunteer work, religious membership, friendship, and parenthood to represent significant and meaningful social roles in their lives.

This article has illustrated that the interrelationships between role occupancy and health among women are complex and depend on life stage as well as on a range of other factors. The article has examined the number of roles occupied; it has not explored women's level of commitment to roles nor the amount of time spent in each role. Nor has it considered the possibility that different roles may have different levels of strains and gratifications that affect their combination.

As Spurlock (1995) argued, multiple roles are a fact of life for women and one that has the potential to provoke conflict, stress, and ill health throughout the lifecycle. At the same time, multiple roles also provide women with multiple sources of satisfaction and achievement. Theories of multiple roles have tended to focus on women of employment age, and there has been a relative neglect of the roles of older women, the contributions they make to society, and the extent to which maintenance of social roles is associated with maintenance of good health. There has also been a neglect of the role of adult developmental processes in women's ability to deal with multiple roles. These data suggest that life stage and ability to cope with multiple roles are complexly related. The challenge is to develop theories that comprehensively deal with multiple roles throughout adult life and that take into account the social and historical factors that affect the relations between role occupancy and health.

REFERENCES

Adelmann, P. K., Antonucci, T. C., Crohan, S. E., & Coleman, L. M. (1990). A causal analysis of employment and health in midlife women. *Women and Health, 16,* 5–20.

Aube, J., Fleury, J., & Smetana, J. (2000). Changes in women's roles: Impact on and social policy implications for the mental health of women and children. *Development and Psychopathology, 12,* 633–656.

Australian Bureau of Statistics. (1997). National Health Survey Australia, 1995: SF–36 population norms. Canberra: Australian Government Publishing Service.

Barnett, R. C., Marshall, N. L., & Singer, J. D. (1992). Job experiences over time, multiple roles, and women's mental health: A longitudinal study. *Journal of Personality and Social Psychology, 62,* 634–644.

Baruch, G. K., & Barnett, R. (1986). Role quality, multiple role involvement, and psychological well-being in midlife women. *Journal of Personality and Social Psychology, 51,* 578–585.

Becker, P. E., & Moen, P. (1999). Scaling back: Dual-earner couples' work-family strategies. *Journal of Marriage and the Family, 61,* 995–1007.

Bell, S., & Lee, C. (2002). Development of the perceived stress questionnaire for young women. *Psychology, Health and Medicine, 7, 189–201.*

Bittman, M. (1992). *Juggling time: How Australian families use their time.* Canberra: Australian Government Publishing Service.

Bromberger, J. T., & Matthews, K. A. (1994). Employment status and depressive symptoms in middle-aged women: A longitudinal investigation. *American Journal of Public Health, 84,* 202–206.

Brooks-Gunn, J., & Chase-Lansdale, P. L. (1995). Adolescent parenthood. In M. H. Bornstein (Ed.), *Handbook of parenting, Vol. 3: Status and social conditions of parenting* (pp. 113–149). Mahwah, NJ: Lawrence Erlbaum Associates, Inc.

Brown, W. J., Bryson, L., Byles, J. E., Dobson, A. J., Lee, C., Mishra, G., & Schofield, M. (1998). Women's Health Australia: Recruitment for a national longitudinal cohort study. *Women and Health, 28,* 23–40.

Brown, W. J., Young, A. F., & Byles, J. B. (1999). Tyranny of distance? The health of mid-age women living in five geographic areas of Australia. *Australian Journal of Rural Health, 7,* 148–154.

Cheung, Y. B. (2000). Marital status and mortality in British women: A longitudinal study. *International Journal of Epidemiology, 29,* 93–99.

Dautzenberg, M. G. H., Diederiks, J. P. M., Philipsen, H., & Tan, F. E. S. (1999). Multigenerational caregiving and well-being: Distress of middle-aged daughters providing assistance to elderly parents. *Women and Health, 29,* 57–74.

Department of Education, Training, and Youth Affairs. (2001). *Students 2000: Selected higher education statistics.* Canberra: Australian Government Publishing Service.

Doress-Worters, P. B. (1994). Adding elder care to women's multiple roles: A critical review of the caregiver stress and multiple roles literatures. *Sex Roles, 31,* 597–616.

Forgays, D. K., & Forgays, D. G. (1993). Personal and environmental factors contributing to parenting stress among employed and nonemployed women. *European Journal of Personality, 7,* 107–118.

Gerson, J. M. (1985). Women returning to school: The consequences of multiple roles. *Sex Roles, 13,* 77–92.

Hibbard, J. H., & Pope, C. R. (1991). Effect of domestic and occupational roles on morbidity and mortality. *Social Science and Medicine, 32,* 805–811.

Home, A. M. (1997). The delicate balance: Demand, support, role strain, and stress in multiple role women. *Social Work and Social Sciences Review, 7,* 131–143.

Home, A. M. (1998). Predicting role conflict, overload, and contagion in adult women university students with families and jobs. *Adult Education Quarterly, 48,* 85–97.

Johnson, N. J., Backlund, E., Sorlie, P. D., & Loveless, C. A. (2000). Marital status and mortality: The national longitudinal study. *Annals of Epidemiology, 10,* 224–238.

Lee, C. (1999). Health, stress and coping among women caregivers: A review. *Journal of Health Psychology, 4,* 27–40.

Lee, C. (2001a). Experiences of family caregiving among older Australian women. *Journal of Health Psychology, 6,* 393–404.

Lee, C. (2001b). Family caregiving: A gender-based analysis of women's experiences. In S. Payne & C. Ellis Hill (Eds.), *Chronic and terminal illness: New perspectives on caring and careers* (pp. 123–139). Oxford, England: Oxford University Press.

Lee, C. (Ed.). (2001c). Women's health Australia: What do we know? What do we need to know? Brisbane: Australian Academic Press.

Lee, C., & Porteous, J. (2002). Experiences of family caregiving among middle-aged Australian women. *Feminism and Psychology, 12,* 79–96.

Lundberg, U. (1996). Influence of paid and unpaid work on psychophysiological stress responses of men and women. *Journal of Occupational Health Psychology, 1,* 117–130.

Martire, L. M., Stephens, M. A. P., & Townsend, A. L. (2000). Centrality of women's multiple roles: Beneficial and detrimental consequences for psychological well-being. *Psychology and Aging, 15,* 148–156.

Mishra, G., & Schofield, M. (1998). Norms for the physical and mental health component summary scores of the SF-36 for young, middle and older Australian women. *Quality of Life Research, 7,* 215–220.

Moen, P., Erickson, M. A., & Dempster-McClain, D. (2000). Social role identities among older adults in a continuing care retirement community. *Research on Aging, 22,* 559–579.

Moen, P., Robison, J., & Dempster-McClain, D. (1995). Caregiving and women's well-being: A life course approach. *Journal of Health and Social Behavior, 36,* 259–273.

Moen, P., & Yu, Y. (2000). Effective work/life strategies: Working couples, work conditions, gender, and life quality. *Social Problems, 47,* 291–326.

Park, J., & Liao, T. F. (2000). The effect of multiple roles of South Korean married women professors: Role changes and the factors that influence potential role gratification and strain. *Sex Roles, 43,* 571–591.

Reifman, A., Biernat, M., & Lang, E. L. (1991). Stress, social support, and health in married professional women with small children. *Psychology of Women Quarterly, 15,* 431–445.

Romans, S. E., Walton, V. A., McNoe, B. M., Herbison, G. P. & Mullen, P. E. (1993). Otago women's health survey 30-month follow-up: I. Onset patterns of non-psychotic psychiatric disorder. *British Journal of Psychiatry, 163,* 733–738.

Roxburgh, S. (1997). The effect of children on the mental health of women in the paid labor force. *Journal of Family Issues, 18,* 270–289.

Spurlock, J. (1995). Multiple roles of women and role strains. *Health Care for Women International, 16,* 501–508.

Stephens, M. A. P., & Franks, M. M. (1999). Parent care in the context of women's multiple roles. *Current Directions in Psychological Science, 8,* 149–152.

Stephens, M. A. P., Townsend, A. L., Martire, L. M., & Druley, J. A. (2001). Balancing parent care with other roles: Interrole conflict of adult daughter caregivers. *Journals of Gerontology Series B, 56,* P24–P34.

Voydanoff, P., & Donnelly, B. W. (1999). Multiple roles and psychological distress: The intersection of the paid worker, spouse, and parent roles with the role of the adult child. *Journal of Marriage and the Family, 61,* 725–738.

Waldron, I., Hughes, M. E., & Brooks, T. L. (1996). Marriage protection and marriage selection: Prospective evidence for reciprocal effects of marital status and health. *Social Science and Medicine, 43,* 113–123.

Waldron, I., Weiss, C. C., & Hughes, M. E. (1998). Interacting effects of multiple roles on women's health. *Journal of Health and Social Behavior, 39,* 216–236.

Wallace, J. E. (1999). Work-to-nonwork conflict among married male and female lawyers. *Journal of Organizational Behavior, 20,* 797–816.

Ware, J. E., & Sherbourne, C. D. (1992). The MOS 36-item short-form health survey (SF–36): I. Conceptual framework and item selection. *Medical Care, 30,* 473–483.

Weatherall, R., Joshi, H., & Macran, S. (1994). Double burden or double blessing? Employment, motherhood and mortality in the Longitudinal Study of England and Wales. *Social Science and Medicine, 38,* 285–297.

Wicks, D., & Mishra, G. (1998). Young Australian women and their aspirations for work, education, and relationships. In E. Carson, A. Jamrozik, & T. Winefield (Eds.), *Unemployment: Economic promise and political will.* (pp. 89–100). Brisbane: Australian Academic Press.

INTERNATIONAL JOURNAL OF BEHAVIORAL MEDICINE, 9(3), 216–227
Copyright © 2002, Lawrence Erlbaum Associates, Inc.

Gender-Specific Association
of Perceived Stress and
Inhibited Breathing Pattern

David E. Anderson and Margaret A. Chesney

Stress can potentiate the development of hypertension via inhibition of renal excretory function. One potential mediating mechanism is an inhibited breathing pattern, because hypoventilation can decrease renal sodium excretion acutely via effects on pCO_2 and acid-base balance. Large individual differences in resting breathing patterns have been well-documented, with some individuals maintaining slow frequency and high pCO_2. Whether this breathing pattern is related to chronic stress has not been investigated. This study reports that high perceived stress over the past month was associated with significantly lower frequency breathing at rest, independently of age, race, or body mass index. This finding was more marked in women than in men. In addition, slow breathing frequency was independently associated with higher resting end tidal CO_2 in both men and women. This is the first known report of an association of sustained stress with an inhibited breathing pattern in humans, and points to a pathway by which chronic stress might contribute to the development of hypertension, especially in women.

Key words: blood pressure (BP), breathing, end tidal CO_2, gender, stress

Behavioral stress can reduce renal excretion of dietary sodium and contribute to the development of hypertension via three physiological mechanisms. First, renal sodium excretion can decrease acutely during behavioral stress that increases renal sympathetic nervous system activity (DiBona & Jones, 1995); increased

David E. Anderson, National Institute on Aging, National Institutes of Health, Baltimore, MD, USA; Margaret A. Chesney, University of California, San Francisco, CA, USA and Office of Research on Women's Health, National Institutes of Health, Baltimore, MD, USA.

Correspondence concerning this article should be sent to David E. Anderson, Laboratory of Cardiovascular Science, National Institute on Aging, 5600 Nathan Shock Drive, Baltimore, MD 21224.

renal sympathetic activity has been implicated in obesity- related hypertension (Hall, Hildebrandt, & Kuo, 2001). Second, behavioral stress can impair renal sodium excretion via increases in pituitary–adrenocortical activity, which stimulates sodium-retaining hormones in the adrenal cortex. For example, this mechanism was proposed to play a role in some forms of experimental hypertension in rodents (Harshfield & Grim, 1997).

A third mechanism by which behavioral stress can impair renal excretory function is suppression of breathing. When respiratory removal of CO_2 is decreased relative to metabolic production, respiratory acidosis occurs; that is, plasma pH decreases. The kidneys respond to decreased plasma pH, not only by reabsorbing buffer compounds (e.g., bicarbonate ions), but also by decreasing sodium and water excretion while increasing excretion of hydrogen ions. Experimental studies showed that voluntary slow frequency breathing sustained at a normal depth was accompanied by a decrease in renal sodium excretion (Anderson, Bagrov, & Austin, 1995) and increases in urinary excretion of endogenous compounds that are sensitive to plasma volume expansion (Bagrov, Fedorova, Dmitrieva, Austin, & Anderson, 1995). In those experiments, the plasma volume remained increased even after plasma pH returned to normal.

In general, breathing adjusts acutely via changes in tidal volume (depth) and/or frequency to match the need of the tissues for oxygen (reviewed by Grossman, 1983). Changes in tidal volume occur in response to changes in metabolic need, being higher during exercise and lower during sleep. By contrast, psychological influences can affect breathing frequency, with increases observed during excitement, and, of particular relevance to this study, decreases during vigilant attention to the environment.

Humans do not all breathe at the same frequency while at rest, but show large individual differences that tend to remain stable over time (Benchetrit et al., 1989). In addition, substantial individual differences in resting pCO_2 are also observed, with individuals who breathe slowly at rest maintaining higher resting end tidal CO_2 than those who breathe more rapidly (Grossman, 1983; Schaefer, 1958). Recent research in our laboratory has found that high resting end tidal CO_2 (PetCO$_2$) is a risk factor for blood pressure (BP) sensitivity to high sodium intake (Anderson, Dhokalia, Parsons, & Bagrov, 1996). In addition, high resting PetCO$_2$ has been found to be an independent correlate of elevated resting systolic blood pressure (SBP), especially in women who are low in trait anger (Anderson, Parsons, & Scuteri, 1999). Thus, chronic hypoventilatory breathing might be a risk factor for some forms of high BP.

Whether individuals who breathe slowly at rest and maintain increased pCO_2 do so in response to chronic stress remains to be investigated. This study hypothesized that high perceived stress in a sample of normotensive men and women is associated with slower frequency breathing at rest than observed in matched controls under low stress. It was also hypothesized that low frequency breathing is associated with a higher resting PetCO$_2$ than high frequency breathing. Finally, high resting PetCO$_2$ was hypothesized to be associated with a higher resting BP in older persons (Scuteri, Parsons, Chesney, & Anderson, 2001). Confirmation of these hypotheses would support the view that behavioral stress can influence renal sodium regulation and BP level via effects on breathing pattern.

METHOD

Participants

The participants were 278 volunteers (151 men, 127 women) from the Baltimore Longitudinal Study on Aging, a multidisciplinary study of normal human aging conducted at the National Institute on Aging. The average age of the women was 57.1 ± 1.4 years and of the men was 58.1 ± 1.5 years. Twenty four percent of the male sample and 32% of the female sample was African American. No significant differences were observed between White and African American women or men in age. The participants were predominantly college-educated, and visited the Gerontology Research Center at approximately 2-year intervals. Each visit includes 2.5 days of evaluation and testing, which includes a physical examination by a healthcare provider; an inventory of medications used; and an intensive set of medical, physiological, and psychological examinations.

Exclusion criteria for this study included a history of stroke, cardiac or pulmonary disease, renal disease, diabetes, or treatment with diuretics, bronchodilators, nonsteroidal anti-inflammatory drugs, psychoactive medication, a history of cigarette smoking within the past year, or estrogen replacement therapy. The study was approved by the Institutional Review Board of The Johns Hopkins University School of Medicine.

Apparatus and Procedures

All participants were studied individually in the afternoon at least 2 hr after the previous meal. Following a description of the purpose of the study and obtaining informed consent, the participant was seated in a reclining chair in a testing room for 25 min. PetCO$_2$ was monitored continuously over this period via a nasal cannula attached to a respiratory gas monitor (Ohmeda, Model 5250, Denver, CO). The participant was instructed to breathe through the nose and an investigator was present in an adjoining room to remind the participant as needed. Peak concentrations of expired CO$_2$ in each breath were digitized and recorded in a dedicated computer (NEC Corporation, Model 3FGe, Santa Clara, CA). The respiratory gas monitor was calibrated before each session with a cannister of 6% CO$_2$. Breathing frequency was also estimated from the respiratory gas monitor. Total breathing frequencies assessed from the respiratory gas monitor in this study are higher than those observed in previous studies from this laboratory (Anderson, Austin, & Haythornthwaite, 1993) and others (Cohn et al., 1982) using inductive plethysmography. This is because the sensitivity of the device to partial breaths is greater than in other methods. However, there is no reason to suspect that any differences between groups would result from the instrument used to measure breathing.

SBP and diastolic blood pressure (DBP) were monitored every 5 min via an occlusion cuff around the nonpreferred arm attached to an oscillometric device (Physiocontrol Lifestat 200, Redmond, WA) and means of the last four measures were determined. Body mass index (BMI) was calculated as weight in kg divided by height in cm^2.

The Perceived Stress Scale (PSS) assesses the degree to which participants perceive the demands of the environment over the previous month as stressful, exceeding their capacity to cope. This scale correlates well with measures of stressful life events (Cohen, Kamarck, & Murmelstein, 1983) and predicts a range of health-related outcomes thought to be associated with appraised stress (Cohen & Williamson, 1988). The 10-item form of this scale was used, which has a coefficient alpha reliability of .78. A total score was derived by summation of the ratings for each question on a 5-point scale.

Data Analysis

Means and standard errors of age, BMI, perceived stress, breathing frequency, $PetCO_2$, SBP and DBP, and heart rate (HR) were calculated separately for men and women, and the significance of the difference was analyzed by two-tailed t tests. Analysis of variance was used to test (a) the significance of the differences in resting breathing frequency between high, medium, and low perceived stress and (b) the significance of the differences in resting $PetCO_2$ between high, medium, and low frequency breathing, separately for men and women. Linear regression analyses were performed to assess the significance of the univariate and stepwise multivariate associations between perceived stress; breathing frequency; end tidal CO_2; and SBP and DBP as a function of age, race, and BMI. All analyses were performed using SPSS software.

RESULTS

Group Characteristics and Univariate Associations

Table 1 shows that resting HR of women was higher than that of men ($p < .001$). No significant differences between genders were observed for any other measures, although the difference between women and men in perceived stress approached significance ($p < .08$).

TABLE 1
Means and Standard Deviations of Characteristics for Women and Men

Variable	Women[a]		Men[b]	
	M	SD	M	SD
Age	57.1	1.4	58.1	1.5
Body mass index (kg/m²)	26.5	0.4	27.3	0.4
Perceived stress score	11.3	0.4	10.2	0.5
Breathing frequency (breaths/min)	19.5	0.3	19.6	0.3
$PetCO_2$ (mmHg)	36.5	0.3	36.4	0.3
Systolic blood pressure (mmHg)	125.1	1.3	125.6	1.2
Diastolic blood pressue (mmHg)	71.8	0.7	74.3	0.9
Heart rate (bpm)	74.8	0.8	69.4	1.0

[a]$n = 151.$ [b]$n = 127.$
*$p < .05.$

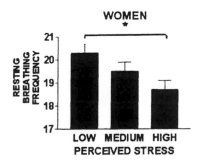

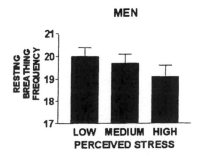

FIGURE 1   Means and standard errors of resting, breathing frequency (breaths/min) for women and men in the upper, middle, and lower tertiles of poerceived stress.

220

For women, the univariate associations of perceived stress with both breathing frequency ($r = -19; p < .05$) and resting $PetCO_2$ ($r = +.16; p < .05$) were significant, but those with age, race, and BMI were not. For men, perceived stress was inversely correlated with age ($r = -.19; p < .05$), but was not significantly associated with race, BMI, breathing frequency, or $PetCO_2$.

Association of Perceived Stress and Breathing Frequency

Figure 1 shows means and standard errors of breathing frequency for women and men under low, medium, and high perceived stress. Women under high stress had significantly slower breathing frequency at rest than women under low stress, $F(2, 145 = 3.78; p < .013)$. Men under high stress showed a nonsignificant trend in the same direction.

TABLE 2
Significant Independent Predictors of Breathing Frequency From Among
Perceived Stress, Age, Race, and Body Mass Index (BMI)

	χ	t	p
Women			
Age (years)	.040	2.71	.008
Perceived stress	− .094	− 2.18	.031
$F_{2,148} = 6.35; p < .002; r^2 = .079$			
Men			
BMI (kg/m²)	.144	2.40	.018
$F_{1,125} = 5.76; p < .018; r^2 = .044$			

TABLE 3
Significant Independent Predictors of End Tidal CO_2 (mmHg) from
Among Breathing Frequency, Age, Race, and Body Mass Index

	c	t	p
Women			
Breathing frequency	−.080	− 2.72	.007
Age (years)	−.015	− 2.40	.018
African American race	.506	2.00	.047
$F_{3,147} = 6.89; p < .000; r^2 = .123$			
Men			
Age (years)	−.283	− 7.39	.000
Breathing frequency	−.117	− 3.03	.003
African American race	1.78	2.83	.005
$F_{3,123} = 31.0; p < .000; r^2 = .430$			

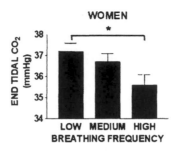

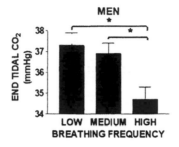

FIGURE 2   Means and standard errors of end tidal CO_2 (PetCO$_2$ in mmHg) for women and men in the upper, middle, and lower tertiles of breathing frequency.
*$p < .05$.

TABLE 4
Multiple Linear Regression Analyses of Predictors of Systolic Blood Pressure (SBP) and Diastolic Blood Pressure (DPB) for 121 Women and 105 Men Over Age 40

	c	t	p
SBP			
Women			
Age (years)	.444	4.70	.000
PetCO (mmHg)	.864	.2.03	.044
	$F_{1,129} = 18.3; p < .000; r^2 = .153$		
Men			
BMI (kg/m²)	.726	2.88	.005
	$F_{1,125} = 8.3; p < .005; r^2 = .055$		
DBP			
Women			
BMI (kg/m²)	.411	2.22	.028
	$F_{1,128} = 4.93; p < .028; r^2 = .037$		
Men			
BMI (kg/m²)	5.45	2.37	.019
	$F_{1,125} = 5.6; p < .019; r^2 = .035$		

Note.   BMI = body mass index.

Table 2 shows the results of multiple regression of perceived stress, age, race, and BMI on breathing frequency for women and men. Perceived stress and age were significant independent predictors of breathing frequency in women, but only BMI was an independent correlate of breathing frequency in men.

Association of Breathing Frequency and End Tidal CO_2

Figure 2 shows means and standard errors of resting $PetCO_2$ for women and men with low, medium, and high breathing frequencies. For both women, $F(2,148 = 3.51; p < .016)$ and men, $F(2, 128 = 5.75; p < .004)$, slower breathing was associated with higher resting $PetCO_2$.

Table 3 shows the results of multiple regression of breathing frequency, age, race, and BMI on $PetCO_2$ for women and men. Breathing frequency, age, and race were significant independent predictors of $PetCO_2$ in women, whereas age, race, and breathing frequency were independent correlates in men.

Association of End Tidal CO_2 and SBP in Older Persons

Table 4 shows the results of multiple regression analyses of $PetCO_2$, age, race, and BMI on SBP and DBP on 121 women and 105 men over age 40. Age and resting $PetCO_2$ were positive independent correlates of resting SBP in women. Table 4 also shows that only BMI was an independent determinant of DBP in women, and of SBP and DBP in men.

DISCUSSION

This is the first known finding of a significant association between high perceived stress and low breathing frequency in women. In addition, low breathing frequency was associated in both women and men with high resting $PetCO_2$, which was previously found to be a risk factor for sodium sensitivity (Anderson et al., 1996) and elevated resting BP in older persons (Anderson et al., 1999). Finally, this study also confirmed the association of high $PetCO_2$ and BP in older women with a new sample.

The finding that high perceived stress is accompanied by low breathing frequency may seem counterintuitive, because emotional arousal (e.g., anxiety or anger) is normally associated with sympathetic nervous system activation, increased breathing, and decreased $PetCO_2$ (Ley & Yelich, 1998; Roth, Wilhelm, & Trabert, 1998). In addition, meditative relaxation can decrease breathing frequency as part of a decreased sympathetic nervous system arousal (e.g., Jevning, Wallace, &

Beidebach, 1992). It would be even more counterintuitive to conclude, however, that a subnormal breathing frequency represents a relaxed state, because ventilation is accomplished with maximum lung efficiency at an optimal frequency with varying tidal volume (Otis, 1964).

An effect of breathing inhibition under stress could be the redistribution of blood flow to the brain that can facilitate vigilant attention to the environment (Mithoefer, 1964). If sustained, this vigilance state could participate in the development of certain forms of hypertension. Although emotional arousal (e.g., job stress) can increase BP acutely (Pickering et al., 1996), chronic hypertension has often been associated with the absence of anger or anxiety (Jorgenson, Johnson, Kolodziej, & Schreer, 1996; Suls, Wan, & Costa, 1995). Clinical observation indicates that hypertensive patients are characterized by psychological defenses that can suppress conscious awareness of negative emotions such as would normally be elicited by existing conditions (Mann, 2000). For example, recent studies have shown that defensiveness, as assessed by the Marlowe–Crowne Scale of Social Desirability, is higher in hypertensive than in normotensive participants (Mann & James, 1998), and is higher in normotensive individuals who go on to develop hypertension than in those who do not (Rutledge & Linden, 2000). Moreover, hypertensive patients are often characterized by alexithymia, a defect in the ability to experience or express emotion (Jula, Salminen, & Saarijarvi, 1999).

The PSS used in this study provided a measure of the extent to which individuals felt their environments over the past month had been unpredictable, uncontrollable, or overwhelming (Cohen, Tyrrell, & Smith, 1991). An advantage of this scale is that its content is independent of specific situations, thus minimizing potential confounding by personal history and interpretation of event significance. An uncontrollable environment could be identified as a state of "hopelessness," as was found to be an independent predictor of hypertension in one recent prospective study (Everson, Kaplan, Goldberg, & Salonen, 2000). In this view, an inhibited breathing pattern would not be merely a transient response to an acute stressor, but a generalized breathing habit conditioned to the assessment that the world is a difficult or dangerous place.

The reasons for the gender difference in the association of perceived stress with breathing frequency remain to be clarified. It has been proposed that women and men respond differently to psychosocial stress, with men more likely than women to show "fight or flight" (Taylor et al., 2000). The literature supports the view that women respond to various stressors with less sympathetic influence on BP and greater parasympathetic influence on HR than men (e.g., Barnett et al., 1999; Frankenhauser, Dunne, & Lundberg, 1976; Lawler, Wilcox, & Anderson, 1995). Gender-specific hormonal influences may also be relevant. Estrogen is known to decrease PetCO$_2$ (Regensteiner et al., 1989), whereas testosterone is a stimulant for the renin-angiotensin system (Reckelhoff, 2001). After menopause, however, the incidence of hypertension increases in women, equal to or surpassing that observed in men (Burt et al., 1995).

Apneic and hypopnic breathing during sleep have been associated with increased daytime pCO_2 (Gold, Schwartz, Wise, & Smith, 1993) and increased prevalence of hypertension (Newman et al., 2001; Ohayon, Guilleminault, Priest, Zulley, & Smirne, 2000). Among hypertensive patients, the prevalence of sleep apnea is greater in women than in men (Silverberg, Oksenberg, & Iaina, 1997), and the extent to which apnea is produced by mechanical obstruction of the airway is less in women than in men (Mohsenin, 2001). However, sleep apnea occurs in less than 5% of the population (Lavie, Silverberg, Oksenberg, & Hoffstein, 2001), and many individuals without sleep apnea maintain resting pCO_2 as high as that observed in those with sleep apnea. Thus, factors other than sleep apnea must account for the high daytime pCO_2 in some persons. This study suggests that conditioned breathing pattern during the daytime could contribute. By contrast, established hypertension has been associated with a mild hyperventilatory breathing pattern (Somers, Mark, Zavala, & Abboud, 1989), which might contraindicate a role for inhibited breathing in its development. However, mechanisms mediating the development of a disorder are not necessarily the same as the organismic adaptations to it.

One limitation of this study is the finding that, although a significant univariate association between perceived stress and $PetCO_2$ was observed in women, that association was not significant in the multivariate analysis. However, breathing frequency and $PetCO_2$ share variance, and the association between perceived stress and breathing frequency may have obscured the association that was observed when breathing frequency was not entered into the analysis.

In conclusion, this study shows that high perceived stress is associated with an inhibited breathing pattern in women that can impact on renal sodium and BP regulation. These findings fit into an emerging literature regarding gender differences in cardiovascular responses to stress. Additional studies are needed to explore the extent to which psychological states, such as defensiveness or hopelessness, that are predictive of future hypertension, are functionally related to the inhibited breathing pattern and high resting $PetCO_2$.

REFERENCES

Anderson, D. E., Austin, J., & Haythornthwaite, J. A. (1993). Blood pressure during sustained inhibitory breathing in the natural environment. *Psychophysiology, 30,* 131–137.

Anderson, D. E., Bagrov, A. Y., & Austin, J. L. (1995). Inhibited breathing decreases renal sodium excretion. *Psychosomatic Medicine, 57,* 373–380.

Anderson, D. E., Dhokalia A., Parsons, D. J., & Bagrov, A. Y. (1996). End tidal CO_2 association with blood pressure response to sodium loading in older adults. *Journal of Hypertension, 14,* 1073–1079.

Anderson, D. E., Parsons, D. J., & Scuteri, A. (1999). End tidal CO_2 is an independent determinant of systolic blood pressure in women. *Journal of Hypertension, 17,* 1073–1079.

Bagrov, A. Y., Fedorova, O. V., Dmitrieva, R. I., Austin, J. L., & Anderson, D. E. (1995). Endogenous marinobufagenin-like immunoreactive factor and Na, K–ATPase inhibition during voluntary hypoventilation. *Hypertension, 26,* 781–788.

Barnett, S. R., Morin, R. J., Kiely, D. K., Gagnon, M., Azhar, G., Knight, E. L. (1999). Effects of age and gender on autonomic control of blood pressure dynamics. *Hypertension, 33,* 1195–1200.

Benchetrit, G., Shea, S. A., Dinh, T. P., Bodocco, S., Baconnier, P., & Guz, A. (1989). Individuality of breathing patterns in adults assessed over time. *Respiratory Physiology, 75,* 199–209.

Burt, V. L., Whelton, P., Roccella, E. J., Brown, C., Cutler, J. A., Higgins, M., Horan M.J., &Labarthe D. (1995). Prevalence of hypertension in the U.S. adult population: Results from the Third National Health and Nutrition Examination Survey, 1988–1991. *Hypertension, 25,* 305–313

Cohen, S., Kamarck, T., & Mermelson, R. (1983). A global measure of perceived stress. *Journal of Health and Social Behavior, 24,* 385–396.

Cohen, S., & Williamson, G. M. (1988). Perceived stress in a probability sample of the United States. In S. Spacapan & S. Oskamp (Eds.), *The social psychology of health* (pp. 31–67). Newbury Park, CA: Sage.

Cohen, S., Tyrell, D. A. J., & Smith, A. P. (1991). Psychological stress and susceptibility to the common cold. *The New England Journal of Medicine, 325,* 606–612.

Cohn, M. A., Rao, A. S., Broudy, M., Birch, S., Watson H., Atkins, N., Davis B., Stoh F.D. (1982). The respiratory inductive plethysmograph: A new non-invasive monitor of respiration. *Bulletin of European Pathophysiological Response, 18,* 643–658.

DiBond, G. F., & Jones, S. Y. (1995). Analysis of renal sympathetic nerves responses to stress. *Hypertension, 25,* 531–538.

Everson, S. A., Kaplan, G. A., Goldberg, D. E., & Salonen, J. T. (2000). Hypertension incidence is predicted by high levels of hopelessness in Finnish men. *Hypertension, 35,* 561–567.

Frankenhauser, A., Dunne, E., & Lundberg, U. (1976). Sex differences in sympathetic-adrenal medullary reactions induced by different stressors. *Psychopharmacology, 47,* 1–5.

Gold, A. R., Schwartz, A. R., Wise, R. A. & Smith, P. L. (1993). Pulmonary function and respiratory chemosensitivity in moderately obese patients with sleep apnea. *Chest, 105,* 1325–1329.

Grossman, P. (1983). Respiration, stress, and cardiovascular function. *Psychophysiology, 20,* 284–299.

Hall, J. E., Hildebrandt, D. A. & Kuo, J. (2001). Obesity hypertension: Role of leptin and sympathetic nervous system. *American Journal of Hypertension, 14,* 103S–115S.

Harshfield, G. A., & Grim, C. E. (1997). Stress hypertension: The "wrong" genes in the "wrong" environment. *Acta Physiological Scandanavia, 640,* 129–132.

Jevning, R., Wallace, R. K., & Beidebach, M. (1992). The physiology of medication: A review. A wakeful hypometabolic integrated response. *Neuroscience and Biobehavioral Reviews, 16,* 415–424.

Jorgenson, R. S., Johnson, B. T., Kolodzeij, M. E., & Schreer, G. E. (1996). Elevated blood pressure and personality: A meta-analytic review. *Psychological Bulletin, 120,* 293–320.

Jula, A., Salminen, J. K., & Saarijarvi, S., (1999). Alexithymia: A facet of essential hypertension. *Hypertension, 33,* 1057–1061.

Lavie, P., Silverberg, D., Oksenberg, A., & Hoffstein, V. (2001). Obstructive sleep apnea and hypertension: From correlative to causative relationship. *Journal of Clinical Hypertension, 3,* 296–301.

Lawler, K., Wilcox Z. C., & Anderson, S. F. (1995). Gender differences in patterns of dynamic cardiovascular regulation. *Psychosomatic Medicine, 57,* 357–365.

Ley, R., & Yelich, G. (1998). Fractional end tidal CO_2 as an index of the effects of stress on math performance and verbal memory of test anxious adolescents. *Biological Psychology, 49,* 83–94.

Mann, S. J. (2000). The mind/body link in essential hypertension: Time for a new paradigm. *Alternative Therapies, 6,* 39–45.

Mann, S. J., & James, G. D. (1998). Defensiveness and essential hypertension. *Journal of Psychosomatic Research, 45,* 139–148.

Mithoefer, J. C. (1964). Breath-holding. In W. O. Fenn & H. Rahn (Eds.), *Handbook of physiology* (pp. 1011–1025). Washington, DC: American Physiological Society.

Mohsenin, V. (2001). Gender differences in the expression of sleep-disordered breathing: Role of upper airway dimensions. *Chest, 120,* 1442–1447.

Newman, A. B., Nieto, F. J., Guidry, U., Lind, B. K., Redline, S., Pickering, T. G., & Quan, S. F. (2001). Relation of sleep-disordered breathing to cardiovascular disease risk factors: the Sleep Heart Health Study. *American Journal of Epidemiology, 154,* 50–59.

Ohayon, M. M., Guilleminault, C., Priest, R. G., Zulley, J., & Smirne, S. (2000). Is sleep- disordered breathing an independent risk factor for hypertension in the general population (13,507 subjects)? *Journal of Psychosomatic Research, 48,* 593–601.

Otis, A. B. (1964). The work of breathing. In W. O. Fenn & H. Rahn (Eds.), *Handbook of physiology* (pp. 463–476). Washington, DC: American Physiological Society.

Pickering, T. G., Devereux, R. B, James, G. D., Gerin, W., Landsbergis, P., Schnall, P. L., Schwartz J. E. (1996). Environmental influences on blood pressure and the role of job strain. *Journal of Hypertension, 14,* S179–S185.

Reckelhoff, J. R. (2001). Gender differences in the regulation of blood pressure. *Hypertension, 37,* 1199–1208.

Regensteiner, J. G., Woodard, W. D., Hagerman, D. D., Weil, J.V., Pickett, C. K., Bender, P. R., & Moore, L. G. (1989). Combined effects of female hormones and metabolic rate on ventilatory drives in women. *Journal of Applied Physiology, 66,* 808–813.

Roth, W. T., Wilhelm, F. H., & Trabert, W. (1998). Voluntary breath holding in panic and generalized anxiety disorders. *Psychosomatic Medicine, 60,* 671–679.

Rutledge, T., & Linden, W. (2000). Defensiveness status predicts 3-year incidence of hypertension. *Journal of Hypertension, 18,* 153–159.

Schaefer, K. E. (1958). Respiratory pattern and respiratory response to CO_2. *Journal of Applied Physiology, 13,* 1–14.

Scuteri, A., Parsons, D. J., Chesney, M. A., & Anderson, D. E. (2001). Anger inhibition potentiates the association of high end tidal CO_2 with blood pressure in women. *Psychosomatic Medicine, 63,* 470–475.

Silverberg, D. S., Oksenberg, A., & Iaina, A. (1997). Sleep related breathing disorders are common contributing factors to the production of essential hypertension but are neglected, underdiagnosed, and undertreated. *American Journal of Hypertension, 10,* 1319–1325.

Somers, V. K., Mark, A. L., Zavala, D. C., & Abboud, F. M. (1989). Contrasting effects of hypoxia and hypercapnia on ventilation and sympathetic activity in humans. *Journal of Applied Physiology, 67,* 2101–2106.

Suls, J., Wan, C. K., & Costa, P. T. (1995). Relationship of trait anger to blood pressure: A meta-analysis. *Health Psychology, 14,* 444–456.

Taylor, S. E., Klein, L. C., Lewis, B. P., Gruenewald, T. L., Gurung, R. A. R., & Updegraff, J. A. (2000). Biobehavioral responses to stress in females: Tend and befriend, not fight or flight, *Psychological Review, 107,* 411–429.

INTERNATIONAL JOURNAL OF BEHAVIORAL MEDICINE, 9(3), 228–242

Women's Hearts Need Special Treatment

Gunilla Burell and Brittmarie Granlund

Coronary heart disease (CHD) is the leading cause of death for both men and women in the Western world. Some studies show that the observed decline in cardiovascular mortality is not as pronounced among women as among men. There is a growing awareness that most earlier studies both on primary and secondary risk factors, diagnosis, prognosis, and rehabilitation have focused mainly on men. Thus, there is a need to develop knowledge about women with CHD and to address gender issues in treatment and rehabilitation strategies. Negative affect and emotions increase risk and may interfere with effective cardiac rehabilitation. Therefore, methods for coping with emotional stress need to be included in treatment regimens after a coronary event. The feasibility of a stress management program for women with CHD was assessed in a pilot study. The program consisted of twenty 2-hr group sessions during 1 year, with 5 to 9 participants per group. The pilot study showed that this treatment program had a low dropout rate and resulted in improvement in quality of life and reduction in stress and symptoms. Further work to optimize psychosocial interventions for women with CHD is needed.

Key words: coronary heart disease (CHD), cardiac rehabilitation, psychosocial intervention, stress management, gender differences, women

"Men die—women suffer." Women in Western countries seek more medical treatment, use more medication, and live longer than men. But they live with greater disability (Grossi, Soares, & Lundberg, 2000). Cardiovascular disease is the leading cause of death for women in the Western world. Although there has been a decline in cardiovascular mortality due to substantial improvements in surgical interven-

Gunilla Burell and Brittmarie Granlund, Department of Behavioral Medicine, Umeå University, Umeå, Sweden.
This research was funded by the National Board of Health and Welfare in Sweden.
Correspondence concerning this article should be addressed to Gunilla Burell, Department of Behavioral Medicine, Umeå University, S–901 85 Umeå, Sweden.

tions and effective medications (Tunstall-Pedoe et al., 1994), this decline is more evident among men than women (Peltonen, Lundberg, Huhtasaari, & Asplund, 2000). There is a growing number of surviving coronary patients living with chronic illnesses such as heart failure, many of whom are older women. This population subgroup has been neglected, relative to younger men. There is a need to improve their care. The purpose of this article is to highlight the need for gender-specific cardiac rehabilitation programs and to present preliminary data on a pilot cardiac rehabilitation program for women.

CARDIAC RISK AND REHABILITATION: GENDER GAPS

Cardiac rehabilitation and secondary prevention programs are to a large extent based on clinical trials of younger male patients. Results have been generalized and applied to women and elderly patients. They have not generally been evaluated for effectiveness in women. *Optimal* treatment is not necessarily *the same* treatment for all.

Increasing evidence points to the importance of depression as an independent risk factor for first and recurrent cardiac events. Numerous studies show that 20% to 40% of coronary heart disease (CHD) patients exhibit depressive symptoms or syndromes (Ahearn et al., 1990; Ariyo et al., 2000; Carney, Freedland, Rich, & Jaffe, 1995; Ferketich, Schwartzbaum, Frid, & Moeschberger, 2000; Ford et al., 1998; Frasure-Smith, Lespérance, & Talajic, 1993, 1995; Horsten, Mittleman, Wamala, Schenck-Gustafsson, & Orth-Gomér, 2000; Ladwig, Roll, Breithardt, Budde, & Borggrefe, 1994). These studies show that depressive symptoms have an adverse impact on prognosis both immediately after a cardiac event (Frasure-Smith et al., 1993, 1995) as well as several decades after the event (Ford et al., 1998). Vital exhaustion—a syndrome of unusual fatigue and loss of energy, increased irritability, and depressive symptoms—has also been demonstrated to increase risk of MI (Appels, Golombeckm, Gorgels, De Vreede, & van Breukelen, 2000; Appels & Mulder, 1988) and of recurrent angina pectoris after angioplasty (Mendes de Leon, Kop, de Swart, Bar, & Appels, 1996). "Type D personality" was shown to increase risk of MI (Denollet et al., 1996). This "distress" syndrome entails a cluster of negative affects and social inhibition.

However, these studies have included only, or mostly, men with CHD. It is rare that men and women have been analyzed separately and compared with each other (see, e.g., the review by Brezinska & Kittel, 1995). Thus, the conclusion must be drawn that there is substantial evidence for men that hostility, depression, social isolation, and inability to express feelings and emotions contribute to increased risk of CHD. It has been inferred that such risk factors affect women, too. However, there may be other psychosocial risks for women, of which we have little knowledge so far.

CARDIAC RISK AND REHABILITATION IN WOMEN

Psychosocial Risk Factors for an Initial Coronary Event

The Framingham Study (Haynes & Feinleib, 1980) showed that women of lower socioeconomic status (SES), and who experienced tension, anxiety, suppressed hostility, lack of vacations, and loneliness, were at increased risk of CHD. Housewives were at particular risk and being employed outside the home was protective. However, tension between work demands and personal commitments may increase risk of CHD (Dixon et al., 1991), especially if a woman's boss is nonsupportive (Eaker, 1989). After adjustment for known risk factors, Dixon et al. (1991) demonstrated that incidence of CHD was significantly elevated in women who felt that their professional opportunities had been constrained by personal commitments to husband and children, and that their family was hurt by their job involvement. This points to a major gender role-related difference between men and women: Many women derive self-esteem from relational success and satisfaction, whereas the male role demands vocational and status success.

Hallstrom et al. (1986), in a prospective study, showed passive dependency, neuroticism (i.e., anxiety), and major and minor depression predicted angina pectoris. Findings from a population-based study in Stockholm (The Stockholm Female Coronary Risk Study) showed that although most women were working outside the home, the main stressors were not work-related, but associated with family and marital problems. Both the risk of developing CHD and of suffering a recurrence were elevated in women with family-related problems. The effect of these factors was stronger in women who had poor coping abilities, were of lower SES, were socially isolated, and were depressed. A recent study by Hallman, Burell, Setterlind, Oden, and Lisspers (2001) showed that women were more sensitive to certain stress-related factors than were men. Psychosocial risk factors that were stronger predictors of CHD for women were physical stress reactions, emotional stress reactions, burnout, family relationships, and daily hassles.

The profile that emerges of "coronary-prone" women is the experience of worries, anxiety, depression, exhaustion, burnout, and low self-esteem, in such settings as a lack of perceived support, low status and powerlessness at work, and considerable family stress. What, then, happens after the woman has had her cardiac event?

Prognosis After the Cardiac Event

Female patients with CHD are often diagnosed and treated by different clinical standards than male patients and, in particular, those women with angina pectoris have often been misunderstood, misinterpreted, and misdiagnosed (Ayanian & Epstein, 1991, 1997). Women have worse prognosis after acute myocardial infarction

(MI) even when adjusted for clinical covariates (Marrugat, Gil, & Sala, 1999). Women report greater general morbidity following an MI than men, including more chronic illness, poorer health, and longer period of reduced activity (for an overview, see Brezinska & Kittel, 1995).

Post-MI women are more likely than men to be anxious, dissatisfied with social support (Frank & Barr-Taylor, 1993), and depressed (Horsten, 2000). Schron, Pawitan, Shumaker, and Hale (1991) showed that post-MI women were more limited in social functioning, less satisfied with their current life situations, and reported more emotional and physical stress symptoms than men, regardless of age and severity of disease.

Psychosocial risk factors increase risk of recurrent CHD. Lack of social support (Orth-Gomér, 1998), low SES (Wamala, 1999), and exhaustion (Appels, Falger, & Schouten, 1993) are important risk factors for recurrence. This array of psychosocial stressors tends to cluster in certain groups and may dramatically increase the likelihood of poorer health outcomes. For example, women in Stockholm who experienced both work and family stress had a five-fold increased risk for CHD compared to women who did not have either of these experiences (Orth-Gomér, 2000). A follow-up of 64 women and 315 men in North Sweden after coronary artery bypass graft (CABG) surgery (Lerner, 2000) showed that women were significantly more depressed than men both before and after surgery. Presurgery they did not differ in anxiety; however, postsurgery women were significantly more anxious than men. The overall results showed that the women's quality of life was significantly lower than the men's both before and after CABG surgery. Thus, distress, feelings of inadequacy, and psychosocial stressors related to family demands may interfere with recovery and increase the risk for recurrent CHD.

Rehabilitation

Previous evaluations of gender-mixed programs have revealed that women are less likely to participate in cardiac rehabilitation programs than men following an MI or CABG surgery. They show lower attendance rates and greater dropout rates from such programs (Ades, Waldmann, McCann, & Weaver, 1992; Boogard, 1984; Conn, Taylor, & Abele, 1991; Downing & Littman, 1994; Haskell, 1994; Schuster & Waldron, 1991). Some reasons for the lower participation and attendance in women may include the physicians' lack of recommendation or referral to cardiac rehabilitation, or a dependent spouse at home who may make attendance more difficult. Because women with CHD are generally working in low status occupations, they may have difficulties in taking time off from work. However, when women do participate in cardiac rehabilitation, they have shown to have similar or better improvement (Ades et al., 1992; Cannistra, Balady, O'Malley, Weiner, & Ryan,

1992; Toobert, Glasgow, Nettekoven, & Brown, 1998). Data from an ongoing study in North Sweden featured active personal follow-ups of men and women after their cardiac event (Norrman, 2002). Results indicated that depressed women attended the offered rehabilitation programs to a larger degree than men and nondepressed women. This suggests the value of active personal follow-up of women as a way to maximize adherence to these programs.

The first major psychosocial intervention trial for CHD patients was the Recurrent Coronary Prevention Project (RCPP), in which Friedman and his coworkers demonstrated that reductions of the so-called Type A Behavior Pattern led to significantly decreased risk of subsequent cardiac morbidity and mortality (Friedman et al., 1986). It should be noted, however, that over 90% of the participants of the RCPP were Caucasian men.

Based on the experiences from this intervention, we developed a 1-year group-based treatment, which was evaluated in a randomized Swedish study (Burell et al., 1994), including only men under the age of 65. The results showed that our treatment format was effective in achieving significant reductions of Type A behavior. Results were promising enough for us to try a group-based stress management program with a larger sample of CHD patients (the New Life Trial; Burell, 1996). Our concept of stress management was broadened to not only include impatient time-urgent Type A behaviors but also depression, anxiety, and fatigue. In the New Life Trial, 228 male and 37 female patients (mean age 58 years) who had undergone CABG surgery were invited to participate and were randomized to 1-year group treatment or a usual care control condition. Overall, a follow-up of 5 to 6.5 years showed significant reductions of total mortality and cardiac events for patients who had received group treatment. The number of women was too small, though, to allow a subgroup analysis.

The RCPP and our own studies thus showed that we had developed a stress management program that could significantly reduce recurrence in younger male patients. Powell et al. (1993) showed that the treatment offered in the RCPP had no benefit in terms of clinical endpoints for women. Predictors of mortality in the women were arrhythmias on ECG, being divorced, and the lack of a college degree (probably a marker of financial stress and lack of power and influence at work) and not Type A behavior. Because the diagnostic instrument for assessing Type A behavior relies on nonverbal behaviors showing intensity of voice, gestures, and body motions, a fair guess is that absence of such reactions could possibly indicate depression.

The Montreal Heart Attack Readjustment Trial (M-HART) Study (Frasure-Smith et al., 1997) was a randomized controlled trial aimed at relieving distress, when it occurred, in post-MI male ($N = 903$) and female ($N = 473$) patients. The program included a telephone contact to determine level of stress, and a home-based nursing intervention to alleviate any stress that was detected. The program had no overall effect on cardiac mortality, and only minimal effects on depression and anxiety. For women in the intervention group, though, there was a higher cardiac and all-cause mortality, compared to control women. The authors' conclusion was that the results do not warrant the implementation of this type of psychosocial intervention, because it may possibly be harmful to some women.

The Enhancing Recovery in Coronary Heart Disease (ENRICHD) trial (The ENRICHD Study Group, 2000) was a randomized controlled trial aimed at reducing depression and increasing social support in 2,481 post-MI patients, 44 % of which were women (The ENRICHD Study Group, 2001). The primary outcome variable was total mortality plus nonfatal MI. The program used Beck cognitive therapy (Beck, 1995) to reduce depression and improve social support. Patients were recruited from eight centers across the United States within 28 days of the MI, and those who scored above a certain criterion of depression and/or low social support and who were randomized to the intervention were offered a combined program of individual and group sessions. The groups were gender-mixed. The overall results showed no survival difference between treatment and usual care patients (Powell, 2002). The treatment patients reduced depression scores significantly more than controls, but the clinical difference was small. Control patients showed a substantial spontaneous improvement in depression and social support. A significant Gender × Treatment interaction indicated that the young Caucasian men did significantly better with this treatment. The women in treatment, however, did significantly worse than control women in terms of recurrence. Some factors other than the cognitive treatment could have contributed to this. The men were younger, had less comorbidity, and were more aggressively treated by their cardiologists. The women in intervention were older and had more comorbidity, factors that are known to contribute to increased risk of recurrence (Schneiderman, 2002). Thus, one should be careful in drawing conclusions about the harmfulness of this psychosocial treatment for women. But it did not do them any good. It should be remembered that the clinical population of CHD women is older, shows more comorbidity, and exhibits more psychological and adjustment problems, thus this was a representative sample.

Past studies of cardiac rehabilitation in women are not encouraging. New directions in the treatment of these patients are needed.

WHAT DO WOMEN WITH CORONARY DISEASE NEED?:
CLINICAL OBSERVATIONS

We have had considerable experience observing and working with women who have experienced coronary events. In the New Life Trial, the treatment groups were gender-mixed, but there were generally only 1 to 2 women with 5 to 7 men. In terms of group dynamics, this situation was unfavorable to the women. The women came across as much less assertive than most of the men, and seemed to withhold their own reactions and opinions. They would be supportive of others—especially of the men in the group—at the expense of expressing themselves. Thus, ingrained, submissive gender role behaviors were often automatically activated in the presence of the men, and an important therapeutic target that emerged for women was to improve self-confidence. Thus, there is reason to target low self-esteem and lack of communication and relational skills in "stress management" training.

The women experienced their disease differently from the men. Despite technically successful surgery, some women still experienced angina, which, of course, was a disappointment to them. More women than men had comorbidity with various diseases, such as cancer, arthritis, and chronic pain. Their risk factor burden was often greater, and yet they often had to wait longer for the correct assessment or diagnosis. Most strikingly, many of these women were depressed, anxious, bitter, and frustrated. They did not converse with other people about their disease, and rarely participated in active rehabilitation programs. They would try to avoid involving the families in their worries and concerns, because they did not want to "burden" them, and thus missed obtaining any necessary support. The life areas where they encountered stress and other problems were quite different from those of the men. Women experienced a lack of both physical and psychological well-being.

In summary, our clinical observations in the New Life gender-mixed groups suggested that the psychological and social consequences of suffering an MI or going through CABG are different for men and women. In the groups, it was sometimes difficult to pay enough attention to the unique problems of the women, such as low self-esteem, family-related stress, and severe life events. It seems reasonable that therapeutic efficacy for female patients could be enhanced in single-gender groups. In this setting, problem areas that are shared by many women could be emphasized, and mutual understanding and support could be maximized.

PILOT RESULTS OF A SKILLS DEVELOPMENT PROGRAM FOR WOMEN WITH CORONARY DISEASE

The aim of this treatment was to help women develop coping skills to manage everyday life problems, minimize cardiac symptoms, improve quality of life, and decrease the risk of a recurrent event. Therapeutic targets included anger management, coping with anxiety and depression, increasing self-assertion and self-efficacy, improving communication, handling social roles and burdens, coping with severe life events and grief, and managing medical symptoms.

Before embarking on a randomized clinical trial, we undertook this pilot study to determine feasibility and effectiveness on psychosocial endpoints. The pilot study was a treatment-group-only study of 23 women with CHD, with a mean age of 59 years (range 46–73). The treatment was conducted in groups, the first six of which took place during a 1-month stay at a wellness center where participants were enrolled in a program of change in dietary and exercise habits. The stress management group sessions were added to this pre-existing general program and then continued in outpatient settings for the remainder of 1 year.

Assessments

Assessments were made before treatment and at the 1-year conclusion of treatment. Perceived stress was assessed by The Everyday Life Stress Scale, a self-administered questionnaire consisting of 20 statements referring to stress reactions in everyday life situations (Lindahl, Burell, Granlund, & Asplund, in preparation). The participant responds to each statement on a 4-point scale. Vital exhaustion was measured by the Maastricht Questionnaire (Appels, Höppener, & Mulder, 1987). Quality of Life was measured using the Göteborg Quality of Life Inventory (Tibblin, Tibblin, Peciva, Kullman, & Svärdsudd et al., 1990), which consists of two parts: the Well-Being Scale, which assesses perceived well-being in various areas of life, and a Symptom Scale.

Description of the Program

Structure.   The program consisted of twenty 2-hr sessions over the course of 1 year. Sessions were held weekly for the first 10 weeks. Patients entered the program between 3 to 6 months after the acute coronary event. Treatment groups consisted of 5 to 9 participants. Each session agenda covered a specific theme and was presented using written texts, case illustrations, slides, films, audio and videotapes, and specific exercises. Participants worked with homework assignments between sessions. Relaxation was practiced in each session to increase the probability that it would be applied as a coping technique in everyday situations.

Each group session began with a few minutes of relaxation. Homework assignments were discussed and the group leader and the participants provided feedback. New themes were introduced using factual information, case illustrations, or other exercises. Throughout the treatment, social support from the group was utilized to facilitate therapeutic progress.

Components of the program.   There were five key components of the program:

1. *Education:* The goals of education can be summarized as developing knowledge about: basic anatomy and physiology of the cardiovascular system; manifestations of, and treatment procedures for, CHD; the symptoms and signs of different types of stress reactions; and the relation between stress and CHD.

Homework assignments included booklets about heart and stress and the study of case illustrations, where the participants can identify their own reactions. Of relevance would be discussions on risk factors of particular importance for women, such as anxiety, exhaustion, and marital stress. Each woman was asked to discuss which of the risk factors were relevant and present when she experienced her cardiac event.

2. *Self-monitoring:* The goals of self-monitoring can be summarized as: becoming more alert to bodily signals such as muscular tension, heart rate, and pain; noticing behavioral and cognitive cues; and observing, reflecting, and drawing conclusions about contingencies of behavior. To increase awareness of one's own reactions, case illustrations and audio-visual materials were used and participants practiced systematic observation of specific behaviors, both in themselves and in other people. The use of systematic diaries during extended periods of time was very important. Group processes were used to facilitate disclosure and ensure social support. Of relevance would be the monitoring of situations involving a need for assertion (e.g., in relation to demands from family members or workmates). One example was the woman who had an offer from a female friend to go on a week's vacation but did not dare to ask her husband for fear of his refusal. She worried that it was her total responsibility to care for her disabled son at home.

3   *Skills training:* The goals of skills training were to reduce negative affect by learning to express thoughts and emotions directly, honestly, and in a caring manner; and learning to *act,* rather than merely *react,* to everyday problems of living. Of relevance would be practicing to let go of perfection in household chores, asserting about own needs in the work situation, and communicating to family about finding recreational time for oneself. The group setting can provide a stage for rehearsing the specific situation. The group leader makes use of group processes, support, and modeling, where both the group leader and the other group members become important role models. A booklet of daily behavioral exercises is used throughout most of the treatment period. The focus is on stress situations related to managing the relationship ("say no lovingly").

The woman in the aforementioned example would need to practice assertive communication with her husband. In this particular case, the woman never even mentioned the issue to her husband because of her fear of violent reactions in him. After having reflected on pros and cons in the group, she decided to decline her friend's offer in order not to provoke her husband. She is one of many examples of the kinds of marital stress that many CHD women encounter, including having to deal with abuse and severe physical or mental illness in family members. Applying certain behaviors that seem appropriate (at least to the group leader!) might in some complex social contexts entail negative consequences. It is important then to agree on what is possible and feasible for the woman to do, and sometimes the first steps toward assertion and self-esteem must be very small and applied with care, persistence, and a long-term perspective.

4. *Cognitive restructuring:* The goals of cognitive restructuring can be summarized as the development of self-talk that enhances self-respect and self-esteem; the ability to cope with the unexpected; tolerance, acceptance, and respect for people different from oneself; trust in others; and positive emotions such as joy, enthusiasm, curiosity, optimism, and love. The contents are the women's personal, day-to-day experiences. Group discussions and sharing of similar experiences facilitate re-interpretation and alternative attributions. Social support and feedback from other group members, who may provide different views and attitudes, helps the participants to adopt alternative ways of thinking.

A relevant example came from one group member who struggled with anginal pains whenever she cleaned her windows. The group members discussed various practical solutions, implying that she could let go of her expectation of doing the work herself. But the woman was resistant and what became obvious was that not being able to clean her house triggered a loss of self-esteem and worth. A situation that may at first glance look trivial could then be used to get at profound issues of re-orientation and finding a new basis for self-esteem. In women's groups, self-monitoring very often reveals situations that many men would regard as trivial, but which often hold a deeper meaning for the woman. The group leader must be sensitive to when this is the case, and it would be counter-therapeutic to step into the role of advice giver.

5. *Spiritual development:* The goals for the discussion of spiritual and life values can be summarized as: creating a balance between work, family, health, pleasurable activities, and spiritual interests; finding new interests; developing joy, enthusiasm, and hope; and accepting and giving love. Spiritual discussions and exercises are an integrated part of the program, especially the last sessions. The social support provided by the group becomes an important facilitating mechanism. In work with women, the issue of—and right to—provide themselves with as much care and need fulfillment as they give to others is crucial.

RESULTS

The results after 1 year of treatment showed significant reductions of self-rated stress ($p < .001$) and vital exhaustion ($p < .01$) and improvements in quality of life ($p < .05$; Table 1).

Attendance was excellent. Once a woman decided to participate in the program, she did not drop out. The mean attendance rate was about 80%.

TABLE 1
Psychological Variables Before Treatment and at Follow-Up

	Pretreatment		Follow-Up		
	M	SD	M	SD	p^a
Everyday life stress	26.2	6.9	16.0	8.0	.000
Vital exhaustion	21.8	6.7	15.0	8.0	.002
GQL well-being	55.4	14.3	61.3	13.9	.045
GQL symptom	13.1	4.9	12.0	6.0	.273

Note. Göteborg Quality of Life Inventory.
[a]Wilcoxon Signed Ranks Tests

DISCUSSION

Our program was feasible and attractive and the dropout rate was low. Thus, it seemed to meet many of the emotional needs of these women. Apparently, when women with CHD are offered rehabilitation programs that are tailored to their needs, good adherence can result. Our initial results suggest that quality of life may improve considerably as well.

Many women were very unhappy when they first came to group sessions. They often blamed themselves for their disease. In contrast, many of our male patients in our former trials (Burell, 1996) seemed to cope fairly well. In our experience, such optimism and eagerness is rare in women with CHD. The women were often worse off medically and might have justification for worry. Very often they were depressed, anxious, and bitter regarding the adequacy of their medical treatment. They felt lonely and had no one to talk to about their situation. They did not want to burden their family and friends. They did not expect people around them to accommodate to their needs in the new situation and/or had difficulties asserting themselves.

Self-worth and communication were core issues in the therapy. At its conclusion, many participants reported that they developed an enhancement of their self-esteem. Many participants expressed what this experience meant to them in the following ways: "I feel calmer; I relax so much better; I worry less; I take it easy. I don't need to finish everything today; I feel hope for the future."

It is clear that this program improved psychosocial function in the women. As we continue our study of it, we will determine whether or not these psychosocial changes translate into improved prognosis.

CONCLUSIONS

We do not yet know how to optimize psychosocial interventions in secondary prevention for women with CHD. Because of this, we believe that it is time we start listening to the women themselves and their common experiences. It is time to start to implement insights into their psychosocial situation after a cardiac event. Some of what has been tried may have been harmful to a number of women. Thus, potential interventions must be relevant not only for women's bodies, but also their psyches and everyday lives. There is a need to offer treatment that attracts women and enhances adherence to treatment. There is a need to meet this imminent challenge, as observed by the U.S. Department of Health and Human Services, National Heart, Lung, and Blood Institute (1995): Further scientific studies should address the following: Evaluations of the effects of cardiac rehabilitation exercise training, education, counseling, and behavioral interventions on special populations. These populations include elderly patients, women of all ages, patients from different ethnic groups, and those with lower educational and socio-economic levels. (Recommendations for additional research).

REFERENCES

Ades, P. A., Waldmann, M. L., McCann, W. J., & Weaver, S. O. (1992). Predictors of cardiac rehabilitation participation in older coronary patients. *Archives of Internal Medicine, 152*(5), 1033–1035.

Appels, A., Falger, P. R. J., & Schouten, E. G. W. (1993). Vital exhaustion as risk indicator for myocardial infarction in women. *Journal of Psychosomatic Research, 37*, 881–890.

Appels, A., Golombeckm, B., Gorgels, A., De Vreede, J., & van Breukelen, G. (2000). Behavioral risk factors of sudden cardiac arrest. *Journal of Psychosomatic Research, 48*(4–5), 463–469.

Appels, A., Höppener, P., & Mulder, P. (1987). A questionnaire to assess premonitory symptoms of myocardial infarction. *International Journal of Cardiology, 17*, 15–24.

Appels, A., & Mulder P. (1988). Excess fatigue as a precursor of myocardial infarction. *European Heart Journal, 9*, 758–764.

Ariyo, A. A., Haan, M., Tangenm C. M., Rutledge, J. C., Cushman, M., Dobs, A., & Furberg, C. D. (2000). Depressive symptoms and risks of coronary heart disease and mortality in elderly Americans. Cardiovascular Health Study Collaborative Research Group. *Circulation, 102*, 1773–1779.

Ayanian J. Z., Epstein A.M. (1991) Differences in the us of procedures between women and men hospitalized for coronary heart disease. *New England Journal of Medicine, 325*, 221.

Ayanian, J. Z., & Epstein, A. M. (1997). Attitudes about treatment of coronary heart disease among women and men presenting for exercise testing. *Journal of General Internal Medicine, 12*, 311–314.

Beck, J. S. (1995). *Cognitive therapy: Basics and beyond.* New York: Guilford.

Boogaard, M. A. (1984). Rehabilitation of the female patient after myocardial infarction. *Nursing Clinical Northern America, 19*, 433.

Brezinska, V., & Kittel, F. (1995). Psychosocial factors of coronary heart disease in women: A review. *Social Science Medicine, 42*, 1351–1365.

Burell, G. (1996). Group psychotherapy in project New Life: Treatment of coronary prone behavior in coronary artery bypass graft surgery patients. In R. Allan & S. Scheidt (Eds.), *Heart & mind: The practice of cardiac psychology* (pp. 291–310). Washington, DC: American Psychological Association.

Burell, G., Öhman, A., Sundin, Ö., Ström, G., Ramund, B., Cullhed, I., & Thoresen, C. E. (1994). Modification of the Type A behavior pattern in post-myocardial infarction patients: A route to cardiac rehabilitation. *International Journal of Behavioral Medicine, 1*, 32–54.

Cannistra, L. B., Balady, G. J., O'Malley, C. J., Weiner, D. A., & Ryan, T. J. (1992). Comparison of the clinical profile and outcome of women and men in cardiac rehabilitation. *American Journal of Cardiology, 69*, 1274–1279.

Carney, R. M., Freedland, K. E., Rich, M. W., & Jaffe, A. S. (1995). Depression as a risk factor for cardiac events in established coronary heart disease: A review of possible mechanisms. *Annals of Behavioral Medicine, 17*, 142–149.

Cohen, S., Mermelstein, R., Kamarck, T., & Hoberman, H. M. (1985). Measuring the functional components of social support. In I. G. Sarason & B. R. Sarason (Eds.), *Social support: Theory, research, and applications* (pp. 73–94). Dordrecht, The Netherlands: Martinus Nijhoff.

Conn, V. S., Taylor, S. G, & Abele, P. B. (1991). Myocardial infarction survivors: Age and gender differences in physical health, psychosocial state, and regimen adherence. *Journal of Advanced Nursing, 16*, 1026–1034.

Contrada, R. J., Hill, D. R., Krantz, D. S., Durel, L. A., & Wright, R. A. (1986, August). *Measuring cognitive and somatic anger and anxiety: Preliminary report.* Paper presented at the Annual Meeting of the American Psychological Association, Washington, DC.

Denollet, J., Sys, S. U., Stroobant, N., Rombouts, H., Gillebert, T. C., & Brutsaert, D. L. (1996). Personality as independent predictor of long-term mortality in patients with coronary heart disease. *Lancet, 347*(8999), 417–421.

Dixon, J. P., Kison, J. K., Spinner J. C. (1991). Tensions between career and interpersonal commitments as a risk factor for cardiovascular disease amoung women. *Women's Health, 17*(3), 33-57.

Eaker E.D. ((1989). Psychosocial factors in the epidemiology of coronary heart disease in women. *Psychiatric Clinics of North America, 12*, 167.

The ENRICHD Study Group. (2000). Enhancing recovery in coronary heart disease (ENRICHD) study: Design and rationale. *American Heart Journal, 139*, 1–9.

Downing J., Littman A. (1994). Gender differences in response to cardiac rehabilitation. In: Czajkowski S.M., Hill D.R., Clarkson T. B. (Eds.) *Women, Behavior and Cardiovascular Disease.* Washingon, DC: NIH Tublications, Vol 94, 3309.

The ENRICHD Study Group. (2001). Enhancing recovery in coronary heart disease (ENRICHD): Baseline characteristics. *American Journal of Cardiology, 88*, 316–322.

Ferketich, A. K., Schwartzbaum, J. A., Frid, D. J., & Moeschberger, M. L. (2000). Depression as an antecedent to heart disease among women and men in the NHANES I study. *Archives of Internal Medicine, 160*, 1261–1268.

Ford, D. E., Mead, L. A., Chang, P. P., Cooper-Patrick, L., Wang, N. Y., & Klag, M. J. (1998). Depression is a risk factor for coronary artery disease in men: The precursors study. *Archives of Internal Medicine, 158*, 1422–1426.

Frank, E., & Barr-Taylor, C. (1993). Coronary heart disease in women: Influences on diagnosis and treatment. *Annals of Behavioral Medicine, 15*, 156–161.

Frasure-Smith, N., Lespérance, F., Prince, R. H., Verrier, P., Garber R. A., Juneau, M., Wolfson, C., & Bourassa M. G. (1997). Randomised trial of home-based psychosocial nursing intervention for patients recovering from myocardial infarction. *The Lancet, 350*(9076), 473–479.

Frasure-Smith, N., Lespérance, F., & Talajic, M. (1993). Depression following myocardial infarction: impact on 6-month survival. *Journal of the American Medical Association, 270*, 1819–1825.

Frasure-Smith, N., Lespérance, F., & Talajic, M. (1995). Depression and 18-month prognosis after myocardial infarction. *Circulation, 91*(4), 999–1005.

Friedman, M., Thoresen, C. E., Gill, J. J., et al. (1986). Alteration of Type A behavior and its effect on cardiac recurrences in postmyocardial infarction patients: Summary results of the Recurrent Coronary Prevention Project. *American Heart Journal, 112*(4), 653–665.

Grossi, G., Soares, J. J. F., & Lundberg, U. (2000). Gender differences in coping with musculoskeletal pain. *International Journal of Behavioral Medicine, 7*, 305–321.

Hallman, T., Burell, G., Setterlind, S., Oden, A., & Lisspers, J. (2001). Psychosocial risk factors for coronary heart disease, their importance compared with other risk factors and gender differences in sensitivity. *Journal of Cardiovascular Risk, 8,* 39–49.

Hallstrom T., Lapidus L., Bengtsson C., Edström K. (1986). Psychosocial factors and risk of ischemic heart disease and death in women: A twelve-year follow-up of participants in the population study of women in Gothenburg, Sweden. *Journal of Psychosomatic Research, 30*(4), 451–459.

Hamilton, M. (1967). Development of a rating scale for primary depressive illness. *British Journal of Social and Clinical Psychology, 6,* 278–296.

Haskell W. L., Alderman, E. L., Fair J. M., et al. (1994). Effects of intensive multiple risk factor reduction on coronary atherosclerosis and clinical cardiac events in men and women with coronary artery disease. The Stanford Coronary Risk Intervention Project (SCRIP). *Circulation, 89*(3), 975–990.

Haynes S. G., Feinleib M. (1980). Women, work and coronary heart disease: Prospective findings from the Framingham heart study. *American Journal of Public Health, 70*(2), 133–141.

Horsten, M., Mittleman, M. A., Wamala, S. P., Schenck-Gustafsson, K., & Orth-Gomér, K. (1999). Social relations and the metabolic syndrome in middle-aged Swedish women. *Journal of Cardiovascular Risk, 6,* 391–397.

Horsten, M., Mittleman, M. A., Wamala, S. P., Schenck-Gustafsson, K., & Orth-Gomér, K. (2000). Depressive symptoms and lack of social integration in relation to prognosis of CHD in middle-aged women: The Stockholm Female Coronary Risk Study. *European Heart Journal, 21,* 1072–1080.

Ladwig, K. H., Roll, G., Breithardt, G., Budde, T., & Borggrefe, M. (1994). Post-infarction depression and incomplete recovery six months after acute myocardial infarction. *Lancet, 343*(8888), 20–23.

Lerner, A. (2000). *Gender differences in quality of life after coronary artery bypass grafting surgery.* Report from the Department of Biomedical Laboratory Science, Umeå University, Sweden.

Lindahl, B., Burell, G., Granlund, B., & Asplund, K. *Gender differences in emotional well-being in a healthy population.* Manuscript in preparation.

Marrugat, J., Gil, M., & Sala, J. (1999). Sex differences in survival rates after acute myocardial infarction. *Journal of Cardiovascular Risk, 6,* 89–97.

Mendes de Leon, C. F., Kop, W. J., de Swart, H. B., Bar, F. W., & Appels, A. P. (1996). Psychosocial characteristics and recurrent events after percutaneous transluminal coronary angioplasty. *American Journal of Cardiology, 77*(4), 252–255.

Norrman, S. (2002, June). Abstract for the VI Nordic Congress on Cardiac Rehabilitation, Reykjavik, Iceland.

Öhman, A., Burell, G., Ramund, B., & Fleischman, N. (1992). Decomposing coronary-prone behavior: Dimensions of Type A behavior in the Videotaped Structured Interview. *Journal of Psychopathology and Behavioral Assessment, 14,* 21–54.

Orth-Gomér, K. (1998). Psychosocial risk factor profile in women with coronary heart disease. In K. Orth-Gomér & M. Chesney (Eds.), *Women, stress, and heart disease.* Mahwah, NJ: Lawrence Erlbaum Associates, Inc.

Orth-Gomér, K., Moser, V., Blom, M., Wamala, S., & Schenck-Gustafsson, K. (1997). Kvinnostress kartläggs. *Läkartidningen, 94,* 632–638.

Orth-Gomér, K., & Schneiderman, N. (Eds.). (1996). *Behavioral medicine approaches to cardiovascular disease prevention.* Mahwah, NJ: Lawrence Erlbaum Associates, Inc.

Orth-Gomér, K., Undén, A-L., & Edwards, M-E. (1988). Social isolation and mortality in ischemic heart disease: A 10-year follow-up study of 150 middle-aged men. *Acta Medica Scandinavica, 224,* 2105–2215.

Orth-Gomér, K., Wamala, S. P., Horsten, M., Schenck-Gustafsson, K., Schneiderman, N., & Mittleman, M. A. (2000). Marital stress worsens prognosis in women with coronary heart disease: The Stockholm Female Coronary Risk Study. *Journal of the American Medical Association, 284,* 3008–3014.

Pearlin, L. I., & Schooler, C. (1976). The structure of coping. *Journal of Health and Social Behavior, 19,* 2–21.

Peltonen, M., Lundberg, V., Huhtasaari, F., & Asplund, K. (2000). Marked improvement in survival after acute myocardial infarction in middle-aged men but not in women: The Northern Sweden MONICA study 1985–1994. *Journal of Internal Medicine, 247,* 579–587.

Powell, L. H., Shaker, L. A., Jones, B. A., Vaccarino, L. V., Thoresen, C. E., & Patillo, J. R. (1993). Psychosocial predictors of mortality in 83 women with premature acute myocardial infarction. *Psychosomatic Medicine, 55,* 426–433.

Powell, L. H. (2002, March). *The ENRICHD clinical trial: Main results.* Paper presented at the annual meeting of the American Psychosomatic Society, Barcelona, Spain.

Schneiderman, N. (2002, March). The ENRICHD clinical trial: Impact on population subgroups. Paper presented at the annual meeting of the American Psychosomatic Society, Barcelona, Spain.

Schron, E. B., Pawitan, Y., Shumaker, S. A., & Hale, C. (1991). Health quality of life differences between men and women in a postinfarction study. *Circulation, 84*(Suppl. II), 245.

Schuster, P. M., & Waldron, J. (1991). Gender differences in cardiac rehabilitation patients. *Rehabilitation Nursing, 69*(16), 248–253.

Tibblin, G., Tibblin, B., Peciva, S., Kullman, S., & Svärdsudd, K. (1990). "The Göteborg Quality of Life Inventory": An assessment of well-being and symptoms among men born 1913 and 1923. *Scandinavian Journal of Primary Health Care* (Suppl 1), 33–38.

Toobert, D. J., Glasgow, R. E., Nettekoven, L. A., & Brown, J. E. (1998). Behavioral and psychosocial effects of intensive lifestyle management for women with coronary heart disease. *Patient Education and Counseling, 35,* 177–188.

Tunstall-Pedoe, H., Kuulasmaa, K., Amouyel, P., Arveiler, D., Rajakangas, A-M., & Pajak, A. (1994). Myocardial infarction and coronary deaths in the World Health Organization MONICA project. *Circulation, 90.*

Undén, A. L., & Orth-Gomér, K. (1989). Development of a social support instrument for use in population surveys. *Social Science Medicine, 29,* 1387–1392.

Wamala, S. P., Lynch, J., & Kaplan, G. A. (2001). Women's exposure to early and later life socioeconomic disadvantage and coronary heart disease risk: the Stockholm Female Coronary Risk Study. *International Journal of Epidemiology, 30,* 275–284.

U.S. Department of Health and Human Services, National Heart, Lung, and Blood Institute. (1995). Cardiac rehabilitation. *Clinical Practice Guideline, 17.*

Wamala, S. P., Mittleman, M. A., Schenck-Gustafsson, K., & Orth-Gomér, K. (1999). Potential explanations for the educational gradient in coronary heart disease: A population-based case-control study of Swedish women. *American Journal of Public Health, 89,* 315–321.

INTERNATIONAL JOURNAL OF BEHAVIORAL MEDICINE, 9(3), 243–262

Relationship Quality Moderates the Effect of Social Support Given by Close Friends on Cardiovascular Reactivity in Women

Darcy Uno, Bert N. Uchino, and Timothy W. Smith

We examined the role of the type of support provided, gender of support provider, and relationship quality in predicting how social support might influence cardiovascular reactivity during acute stress in women. A group of 88 women received either emotional, instrumental, or no support from a close female or male friend while performing a series of speech tasks. Results suggest that the effectiveness of social support for women depended primarily on the quality of the friendship (i.e., purely positive, or ambivalent). More specifically, women who interacted with a female, ambivalent friend had the largest changes in diastolic blood pressure, total peripheral resistance (TPR), and pre-ejection period compared to the other conditions. Furthermore, receiving emotional support from a purely positive friend was related to lower increases in cardiac output (CO) compared to a no-support condition. In contrast, receiving emotional support from an ambivalent friend was related to larger increases in CO and only small changes in TPR when compared to individuals in the no-support condition. These data are discussed in light of the psychosocial processes underlying social support effects in women, and the importance of a more comprehensive view of how close relationships influence cardiovascular function.

Darcy Uno, Bert N. Uchino, and Timothy W. Smith, University of Utah and Health Psychology Program, Support and Reactivity, Salt Lake City, UT, USA.

This research was generously supported by Grant 1 R01 MH58690–01 from the National Institute of Mental Health awarded to Bert N. Uchino.

We thank David Lozano, Daniel Litvack, and John T. Cacioppo for their expert technical assistance and for providing us with copies of their data acquisition and reduction software (i.e., ANS suite). We also thank John T. Cacioppo for his valuable comments on a draft of this article.

Correspondence concerning this article should be addressed to Bert N. Uchino, University of Utah, Department of Psychology, 390 S. 1530 E. Room 502, Salt Lake City, Utah 84112–0251.

Key words: social support, relationship quality, cardiovascular reactivity, womens' health.

There is strong epidemiological evidence linking social support to lower risk for coronary heart disease as well as for morbidity and mortality from all causes (Berkman, 1995; Cohen, S., 1988; House, Landis, & Umberson, 1988). However, little is known about the more specific mechanisms or processes by which social relationships influence long-term health. One promising way to examine such mechanistic questions is illustrated by recent research on laboratory paradigms of social support. Cohen and Wills (1985) proposed a stress-buffering model that suggests psychological stress has pathogenic effects on physiological and health- relevant processes (see Manuck, 1994), and that social support protects an individual from its deleterious effects. Consistent with this stress-buffering hypothesis, laboratory studies have found that the provision of support during stressful tasks decreases heart rate (HR) and blood pressure (BP) reactivity (Lepore, 1998; Uchino, Cacioppo, & Kiecolt-Glaser, 1996). Thus, although other mechanisms are also important (e.g., social control of health behaviors; Umberson, 1987), changes in cardiovascular reactivity represent another potential mechanism linking relationships to health outcomes.

It is important to note that epidemiological studies suggest that the association between social support and health outcomes may be more complex in women (Seeman, 1996; Shumaker & Hill, 1991). For instance, psychophysiological studies suggest that women may be more physiologically reactive during relationship interactions, although the mechanisms responsible for this effect remain to be determined (Kiecolt-Glaser & Newton, 2001). Hence, laboratory studies of cardiovascular responses among women provide an important opportunity to identify contextual factors that could moderate the benefits and costs associated with their social relationships. The primary goal of this study, therefore, was to utilize a laboratory paradigm to test several hypothesized factors that might influence the effectiveness of social support in women based on the larger social support literature. More specifically, this study investigated the impact that (a) the type of support provided by a friend, (b) the gender of the friend, and (c) the quality of the friendship had on changes in cardiovascular reactivity during acute stress.

There are several proposed contextual factors that could alter the impact of social relationships on cardiovascular responses in women. Flaherty and Richman (1989) argued that socialization processes result in women both preferring and benefiting more from the specific dimension of emotional support. Results of their study with medical students provided evidence that women appeared to benefit more from emotional support than other support types. In this study, we tested this proposition as women engaged in a series of speeches while a close male or female friend provided either emotional, instrumental, or no support via handwritten notes. There has been some concern in the prior literature that evaluation apprehension might be particularly strong when the friend is directly visible (Allen, Blascovich, Tomaka, & Kelsey, 1991). Importantly, the use of handwritten notes allowed us to minimize evaluation that could interfere with social support effects.

Gender of the support provider may also play an important role in the association between stress and reactivity in women because of possible differences in the perception and meaning of receiving social support from men versus women. In fact, studies in the stress and coping literature suggest that women are more likely to seek support from a same-sex friend (Barbee, Gulley, & Cunningham, 1990; Burke & Weir, 1978; Flaherty & Richman, 1989). It is therefore possible that women may be more sensitive to the supportive actions of other women (Barbee et al., 1990; Flaherty & Richman, 1989). In a laboratory study using confederates to deliver supportive or neutral comments, support from women attenuated cardiovascular reactivity but support from men did not (Glynn, Christenfeld, & Gerin, 1999). However, the effects of gender of support provider might differ when support is given by an actual network member (e.g., a friend; see Christenfeld et al., 1997).

A third important factor possibly influencing the effectiveness of social support in women may be related to the quality of the relationship. In a recent review of the marital literature, Kiecolt- Glaser and Newton (2001) found that women tend to be more reactive to the quality (especially negative aspects) of the relationship. This is a noteworthy point as many of the predictions from the larger social support and health literature assume that the relationship is one that is characterized predominately by positive feelings. However, not all close relationships are equally supportive. Research suggests that many close relationships are characterized by feelings of both positivity and negativity (Barrera, 1980; Coyne & DeLongis, 1986; Fincham & Linfield, 1997; Rook, 1984; Uchino, Holt-Lunstad, Uno, & Flinders, 2001). However, the implication for this "ambivalence" in close relationships has not been adequately examined as most of the prior research on social support has ignored the negative aspects that may co-occur with the positive aspects of close relationships (Uchino et al., 2001).

We have argued that receiving support within the context of an ambivalent relationship may not be effective in reducing stress because the co-occurring negative feelings can interfere with the supportive communication (e.g., questioning sincerity of support). This would suggest that receiving support from an ambivalent network member may not result in beneficial stress- buffering effects. Furthermore, interactions with ambivalent network members may be generally stressful due to the unpredictability inherent in these relationships. Consistent with this suggestion we have found that older adults with many ambivalent network ties were more depressed and evidenced greater cardiovascular reactivity during stress (Uchino et al. 2001). Thus, although decreased reactivity may be one mechanism by which supportive relationships influence better health outcomes, increased reactivity due to interpersonal stress may be a mechanism linking ambivalent ties to poorer health outcomes.

Due to research suggesting the importance of relationship quality for women, it should be highlighted that this factor should influence the effectiveness of the type of support provided and the gender of support provider in a predictable manner. For instance, because women prefer to seek out support from other women, they may be more sensitive to the quality of the relationship within such interactions (i.e., Gender of Support Provider × Relationship Quality interactions). It is also possible that women may benefit more from emotional support provided by a purely supportive relationship (i.e., Relationship Quality × Support Type interaction). This study will allow us to investigate the more complex processes based on the larger social support literature by which social support may influence reactivity during acute stress in women.

METHOD

Participants and Design

Eighty eight undergraduate women (M age = 21) and one of their male or female friends were recruited from introductory psychology classes and from newspaper advertisements. In return for their participation, students either received $10 or 2 hr of experimental extra credit for their psychology class grades and their friends were compensated $5 for their time.

Participants were randomly assigned to (a) bring in a male or female friend and to (b) one of three support manipulations (no-support, emotional support, instrumental support) so that there were an equal number of male and female friends in each condition. Participants were told to bring in a close, nonromantic friend whom they had known for at least 6 months. The quality of the friendship was assessed via the social relationships index that was used to categorize the relationship as purely positive or ambivalent (see later). Participants then participated in a baseline and a series of speeches during an experimental period. This resulted in a 3 × 2 × 2 (Support Type: No-support, Instrumental Support, Emotional Support × Gender of Friend: Female, Male × Relationship Type: Supportive, Ambivalent) design.

Procedure

On arrival at the laboratory, informed consent was obtained and the participant was asked to fill out a background health questionnaire, had her height and weight recorded on a Health-o- meter scale, and was escorted into a separate sound attenuated room where the BP cuff and physiological sensors were attached (see later). After an adaptation period, the participant was instructed to relax for 10 min while resting measures of cardiovascular function were obtained (Jennings, Kamarck, Stewart, Eddy, & Johnson, 1992). Impedance cardiograph readings were recorded continuously during the last 5 min of the baseline period, and HR and BP assessments were obtained every 90 sec. During that time, the friend was debriefed about the purpose of the experiment and was informed about their role in the study.

The friend was instructed to write supportive notes to the participant to be used during the course of the study. The messages in the notes were identical within each supportive condition. Essentially, the friend was asked to copy the message of a prewritten note onto a piece of paper that would be given to the participant during the speech period. The friend was instructed not to change the message in any way but was asked to personalize the note such that the participant would believe that they wrote the note. To ensure the integrity of the notes, the experimenter checked the messages written.

Following the resting assessment, participants then completed the perceived stress scale (Lepore, Allen, & Evans, 1993). They were then informed that they would be giving three 1-min speeches on current events topics (see Smith, Nealey, Kircher, & Limon, 1997). Participants were instructed to state their opinions on each topic and were asked to speak for 1 min supporting each opinion.

Participants were informed at the beginning of the experiment that their friends would be listening to them give their speeches and whenever possible they would try to send them a note filled with suggestions and/or comments to help and support them through the task. After the preparation period and prior to each speech, the experimenter entered the chamber to give the participant handwritten notes from their friends. Participants received a total of three notes, one prior to each 1-min speech. An example of an emotionally supportive comment was, "I would think that some people are a little nervous doing this, but you are doing just fine." In terms of an instrumentally supportive comment, an example note was, "I was thinking about your topics and jotted down these ideas in support of the statement. Thought they might help you in your speech. For the school uniforms topic, maybe you could say, It would make students take school more seriously because they wouldn't focus so much on what people are wearing." An example of a comment in the no-support condition was "I'm sorry I couldn't think of anything to help you."

Participants were given 3 min to prepare their speech responses. At the end of the preparation period, participants were verbally prompted when to begin and end each speech. Physiological readings were recorded during each of the three speeches. At the end of the speech period, participants were again asked to complete the perceived stress scale, a social support manipulation check (see later), a task engagement measure (Smith et al., 1997), and the interpersonal adjective scale revised (IAS–R; Wiggins, Trapnell, & Phillips, 1988). Finally, participants and their friends were fully debriefed and thanked for their participation in the study.

Measures

Cardiovascular measures.   The Dinamap monitor (Critikon corporation, Tampa, FL) was used to estimate systolic blood pressure (SBP), diastolic blood pressure (DBP), and mean arterial blood pressure (MAP) from the upper nondominant arm using the occillometric method. The BP cuff was positioned on the participant using the proper manufacturer's specifications.

A Minnesota Cardiograph was used to measure ECG, basal thoracic impedance (Z_0), and the first derivative of the impedance signal (dZ/dt). Four mylar bands were placed on the neck and thoracic regions according to published guidelines (Sherwood et al., 1990). A 4 mA AC current at 100 kHz was passed through the two outer bands, and Z_0 and dZ/dt were recorded from the two inner bands. The impedance data were ensemble averaged within 1-min epochs, and each waveform was verified or edited prior to analyses. Stroke volume (SV) was estimated using the Kubicek equation (Sherwood et al., 1990) and then used to compute subsequent cardiac output (CO; i.e., $CO = HR/1000 \times SV$) and total peripheral resistance (TPR; i.e., $TPR = MAP/CO \times 80$). Finally, pre-ejection period (PEP), which sensitively measures sympathetic control of the heart, was calculated as the time interval in ms between the Q-point of the ECG and the B-point of the dz/dt signal.

Respiratory sinus arrhythmia (RSA) provides a noninvasive measure of parasympathetic control of the heart and was calculated based on the digitized interbeat intervals that were checked and edited for artifacts using the detection algorithm of Berntson, Quigley, Jang, and Boysen (1990). After linear detrending, the heart period time series was band pass filtered from .12 to .40 Hz using an interpolated finite impulse response filter (Nuevo, Cheng-Yu, & Mitra, 1984). RSA was then calculated as the natural log of the area under the heart period spectrum (calculated by a Fast Fourier Transform and scaled to $msec^2/Hz$).

Quality of relationship measure.   The social relationships inventory (SRI) was developed as a modified version of the social support interview (Fiore, Becker, & Coppel, 1983; Kiecolt-Glaser, Dura, Speicher, Trask, & Glaser, 1991). Individuals were instructed to rate how helpful and upsetting they feel their friend is when they need social support on a scale ranging from 1 (*not at all*) to 6 (*very much*). The SRI has been found to have good internal consistency and has adequate test–retest reliability and convergent validity (Uchino et al., 2001). For instance, in our prior work with the SRI, the assessment of positivity and negativity for network members was characterized by good internal consistency (alphas of .81 to .87). These network measures of positivity and negativity were also temporally stable with significant 2-week test–retest correlations of $r = .81$ ($p < .001$) for positivity and $r = .83$ ($p < .001$) for negativity.

We operationalized supportive and ambivalent relationships consistent with the procedure of Barrera (1980) and Rook (1984). Thus, a socially supportive network member was an individual rated as greater than "1" on positivity and only a "1" on negativity, whereas an ambivalent network member was an individual rated as greater than "1" on both positivity and negativity. In this study, 44% of the sample had ambivalent relationships (characterized by both positivity and negativity) and 56% had supportive relationships (characterized by only positivity and no negativity) with their friends. This distribution is consistent with our prior work suggesting that ambivalent ties make up almost half of individuals important network members (Uchino et al., 2001). Finally, ancillary questions on the SRI verified the closeness of the friends that provided support in this study. Mean ratings of the importance of their relationship with the friend were high ($M = 4.5$, $SD = 1.05$) on a 6-point scale ranging from 1 (*not at all important*) to 6 (*very important scale*), with an average of 4.4 days ($SD = 1.95$) of contact per week.

Demographic and health measures.   Participants also provided basic demographic information including age, ethnicity, yearly income, and marital status. They were also asked to report health- related information to verify that they were not on any cardiovascular-altering medications.

Manipulation Checks

Social support.   A 10-item questionnaire was designed to assess a participant's perceptions of the social support manipulation. The items on this scale were divided into two scales: emotional support and instrumental support. Examples of items on both of the aforementioned scales are, "My friend had faith in me and my abilities to do the speeches" and "My friend gave me suggestions on what to say for my speeches," respectively. The internal consistency of the emotional support subscale and of the instrumental support subscale was .76. Participants were also asked to make a forced-choice selection in response to the following single-item statement: "During the experiment, my friend was trying to: give me problem focused help, make me feel better, or did neither."[1]

---

[1]The scale items can be obtained by contacting Bert N. Uchino.

IAS–R.   One difficulty in conducting social psychophysiological studies of cardiovascular reactivity is verifying which aspects of the social context are manipulated and assessing the extent of differences on these dimensions (Smith, Limon, Gallo, & Ngu, 1996). We have suggested using the interpersonal circumplex to provide manipulation checks in such studies (Smith, Gallo, Goble, Ngu, & Stark, 1998). This permits useful checks within studies, and affords comparisons across studies (Smith et al., 1998; Smith et al., 1996). Toward this end, an abbreviated version of the IAS–R was used to obtain standardized measures of the participant's construal of their friend's behavior during the experiment (Wiggins et al., 1988). The IAS–R is a widely used self-report measure in which an overall measure of dominance and affiliation can be obtained (see validity data from Kiesler, 1991; Wiggins & Broughton, 1991) and we have found the shortened version sensitive to experimental manipulations of interpersonal processes (Smith, Gallo, & Ruiz, in press). Conceptual and empirical analyses indicate that social support is clearly on the warm/friendly side of the circumplex, although specific supportive behaviors vary in their level of dominance or control (Trobst, 2000).

Perceived stress and task engagement.   Perceived stress was measured using a 6-item bipolar adjective scale (see Lepore et al., 1993). The participant was asked to rate the extent to which they feel stressed–relaxed, uncomfortable–comfortable, anxious–not anxious, not nervous–nervous, calm–excited, and worried–content. Consistent with our prior work, participants were also asked about their level of task engagement (Smith et al., 1997).

RESULTS

Preliminary Analyses

To examine the baseline equivalency between groups, a series of $3 \times 2 \times 2$ (Support Type × Gender of Friend × Relationship Type) analyses of variance (ANOVAs) were performed. Results revealed no main effects or interaction on basic demographic variables such as age, ethnicity, yearly income, and marital status (all $ps >$ .18). No main effects or interactions were found on the perceived stress measure. All in all, results revealed that the groups were comparable on the baseline assessments.

Analyses of the SRI positivity and negativity assessments revealed no main effects or interactions with support type on either dimension. Replicating prior research, women friends were rated as more positive (supportive) than male friends, $F(1, 76) = 4.52, p < .04$. Consistent with our relationship quality classification procedure, ambivalent friends were associated with higher levels of negativity than supportive friends, $F(1, 76) = 76.6, p < .001$. Importantly, ambivalent friends did not differ from supportive friends on levels of positivity ($p > .21$).

Manipulation Checks and Self-Report Measures

Repeated measures ANOVAs were carried out to test if the laboratory stressor was effective. Analyses revealed that the stressor resulted in significant increases in perceived stress, $F(1, 87) = 102.9, p < .001$. Corresponding analyses on the cardiovascular measures revealed that the stress protocol led to increases in SBP, $F(3, 243) = 124.33, p < .001$; DBP, $F(3, 243) = 107.93, p < .001$; CO, $F(3, 258) = 10.64, p < .001$; and TPR, $F(3, 240) = 12.20, p < .001$. The increase in CO was due to a task-related rise in HR, $F(3, 258) = 186.39, p < .001$, as SV declined during the task, $F(3, 258) = 32.83, p < .001$. In addition, PEP was shortened, $F(3, 258) = 62.59, p < .001$, and RSA decreased, $F(3, 258) = 9.61, p < .001$, during the stressors.

A series of $3 \times 2 \times 2$ (Support Type × Gender of Friend × Relationship Type) ANOVAs were run to see if participants were able to recognize the type of support that they received. As expected, a significant support type main effect was found on both the emotional, $F(2, 82) = 75.87, p < .001$, and the instrumental, $F(2, 82) = 121.29, p < .001$, dimensions of the social support manipulation check. As shown in Table 1, follow-up contrasts revealed that individuals in the emotional support condition reported receiving significantly higher levels of emotional support than did individuals in the no-support and instrumental support conditions. In addition, individuals in the instrumental condition reported receiving higher levels of instrumental support than did individuals in the emotional support and the no-support groups. Consistent with prior research, a main effect for gender of friend also revealed that participants rated female friends as being more emotionally supportive than male friends, $F(1, 82) = 9.08, p < .01$.

TABLE 1
Mean Levels of the Manipulation Checks as a Function of Type of Support Received

Measure	Support Condition		
	Emotional	Instrumental	No Support
Emotional support	3.7[b]	2.7[a]	2.1[a]
Instrumental support	2.0[a]	3.1[b]	1.4[a]
IAS-Affiliation	0.4[a]	0.4[a]	−0.8[b]
IAS-Dominance	0.4[a]	0.2[a]	−0.5[b]

Note. IAS = Interpersonal Adjective Scale. Means within rows with different subscripts are significantly different at $p < .05$.

On the forced-choice item of the social support manipulation check, participants were able to accurately identify (93.2%) which condition they were in.

To identify the social context captured by our manipulation, similar ANOVAs were conducted on the IAS–R. As shown in Table 1, significant type of support main effects were found on the affiliation, $F(2, 82) = 17.84, p < .001$, and the dominance, $F(2, 82) = 13.16, p < .001$, dimensions. Participants in the emotional support condition reported significantly higher affiliation and dominance scores when compared with those in the no-support group. Participants in the instrumental support group also had significantly higher affiliation and dominance scores than those individuals who were in the no-support group. The emotional and instrumental support groups did not differ from each other in ratings of affiliation or dominance. Participants also perceived their female friends as being more affiliative than their male friends, $F(1, 82) = 4.35, p < .05$. In summary, these data suggest the effectiveness of the manipulations that were used to test the theoretical predictions of the study.

Consistent with our expectations, several additional findings emerged indicating that women had different experiences as a result of interacting with a particular relationship type. A significant Relationship Type × Gender of Friend interaction was found on the dominance dimension of the IAS, $F(1, 76) = 4.17, p < .05$. Female, ambivalent friends were perceived to be more dominant than supportive female or male friends. In addition, a marginally significant finding emerged on the self-report task difficulty measure, $F(1, 76) = 3.62, p = .06$. Participants who received notes from ambivalent, female friends rated the task to be the hardest when compared to the other friends. These data suggest that the women who received notes from an ambivalent female friend construed the task in a more negative light.

Main Analysis

A series of 2 × 3 × 2 (Relationship Type × Support Type × Gender of Support Provider) analyses of covariance were performed to examine the effect of our variables on physiological responsiveness. The major physiological dependent measures were SBP, DBP, and HR. In addition, because BP and HR are multiply determined cardiovascular endpoints, measures of PEP, RSA, CO, and TPR were also used as dependent variables to better assess the underlying mechanisms responsible for the changes in cardiovascular reactivity across conditions. All physiological measurements were first reduced and averaged into 1-min segments. An average value was then obtained for each epoch to increase the reliability of these assessments (Kamarck et al., 1992). Change scores were then computed to quantify physiological responses (average stress epoch–average baseline epoch), with baseline values statistically controlled in the analyses (Llabre, Spitzer, Saab, Ironson, & Schneiderman, 1991).[2]

Analyses were also conducted considering the potential influence of body mass on cardiovascular reactivity. The results reported in the text are unchanged while statistically controlling for group differences in body mass index.

Our analyses revealed no main effects for the manipulated factors of type of support and gender of support provider on cardiovascular reactivity. However, consistent with our expectations regarding the importance of relationship quality, several main effects for relationship type emerged on the cardiovascular responses of women. More specifically, women interacting with ambivalent friends had significantly greater increases in TPR, $F(1, 74) = 4.40, p < .04$, than women interacting with supportive friends ($M = 358.5$ vs. 161.8 dynes/s). Consistent with this vascular effect, women interacting with ambivalent ties also had marginally higher DBP reactivity, $F(1, 75) = 3.33, p = .07$, compared to those interacting with supportive friends ($M = 15.5$ vs. 12.5 mmHg). In addition, significant statistical interactions emerged in the full factorial analyses for relationship type and gender of friend, as well as relationship type and support type. Means for all cardiovascular measure for the full factorial design are summarized in Table 2.

Relationship Type × Gender of Friend Findings

A number of significant two-way interactions between relationship type and gender of friend emerged in predicting reactivity, including DBP, $F(1, 69) = 4.86, p < .05$. As seen in Figure 1 (top), women who interacted with female, ambivalent friends displayed higher levels of reactivity when compared to those who interacted with female, supportive friends ($p < .01$). The elevated reactivity associated with ambivalent female friends was also significantly different than the reactivity found when interacting with ambivalent male friends ($p < .05$). Subsequent analyses of the underlying determinants of these DBP responses revealed a marginally significant interaction between relationship type and gender of friend on TPR reactivity, $F(1, 73) = 3.30, p = .07$. Follow-up comparisons indicated that women interacting with an ambivalent female friend had greater in-

---

[2]Preliminary analyses revealed several significant interaction involving speech epoch (1st, 2nd, 3rd speech). However, in only one case did the interaction qualify any of the results reported in this article (i.e., Relationship Quality × Support Type × Epoch interaction for TPR; results reported in text became more apparent over time). As a result, we averaged across epochs to increase the reliability of these assessments as recommended by Kamarck et al. (1992). Individuals interested in the results involving each epoch can contact Bert N. Uchino.

TABLE 2

Mean Cardiovascular Changes as a Function of Relationship Type and Support Condition for Male Support Providers and Female Support Providers

| Cardiovascular Measures | Male Friend | | | | | | |
| | Supportive Friend | | | Ambivalent Friend | | | |
	Emotional	Instrumental	No Support	Emotional	Instrumental	No Support	Average
				Male Friend			
SBP	10.4	18.5	17.3	17.7	13.9	13.8	15.3
DBP	11.5	18.7	12.7	14.1	12.8	12.9	13.8
CO	.01	.0	.67	.44	.22	-.28	.18
TPR	316.3	380.2	118.9	135.2	243.5	532.3	287.7
HR	7.5	17.7	14.4	18.5	12.9	9.3	13.4
PEP	-3.2	-12.5	-10.2	-6.1	-9.6	-0.4	-7.0
RSA	-.03	-.50	-.74	-.69	-.5	-.32	-.46
				Female Friend			
SBP	16.5	12.5	14.3	18.5	17.1	16.4	15.9
DBP	11.1	7.8	13.2	15.3	18.1	19.5	14.2
CO	.26	.47	.54	.60	-.14	.02	.29
TPR	310.0	-283.5	112.0	179.4	533.0	553.6	234.1
HR	12.7	11.9	12.1	16.9	16.0	16.1	14.3
PEP	-5.1	-3.3	-7.7	-12.1	-10.4	-12.6	-8.6
RSA	-.41	-.32	-.35	-.65	-.59	-.67	-.50

Note. SBP = systolic blood pressure; DBP = diastolic blood pressure; CO = cardiac output; TPR = total peripheral resistance; HR = heart rate; PEP = pre-ejection period; RSA = respiratory sinus arrhythmia.

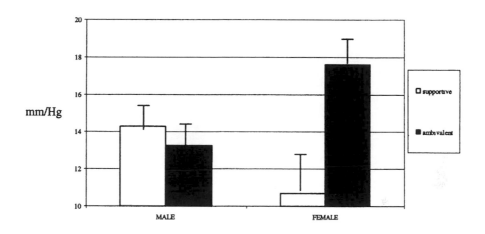

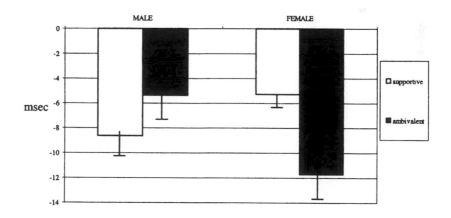

FIGURE 1   Top panel. Gender of friend x relationships type interaction for DBP
reactivity. Bottom panel. Gender of friend x relationships type interaction for PEP reactivity.

crease in TPR ($p < .05$), suggesting a vascular basis for the DBP effect.

Analyses also revealed a significant two-way interaction between gender of
friend and relationship type for PEP, $F(1, 74) = 7.94, p < .01$. Consistent with the
other effects, women who interacted with an ambivalent female friend had a greater
shortening of PEP (indicating greater increases in sympathetic control of the heart)

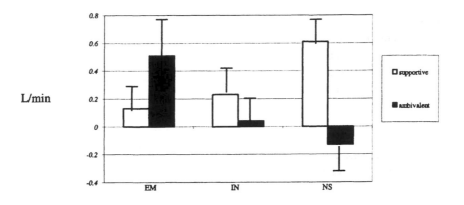

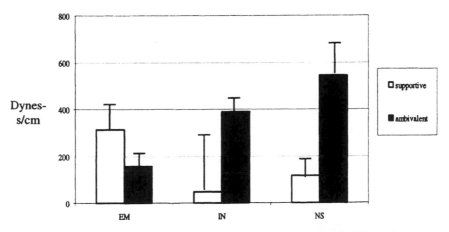

FIGURE 2   Top panel. Type of support x relationships type interaction for CO reactivity. Bottom panel. Gender of friend x relationships type interaction for PEP reactivity.

than those interacting with either a supportive female friend ($p = .01$) or an ambivalent male friend ($p = .08$; see Figure 1, bottom).

Relationship Type × Support Type Findings

Analyses of CO revealed a significant two-way interaction between relationship type and support type, $F(2, 74) = 4.12, p < .05$; see Figure 2, top. Simple effects analyses revealed that the main effect for support type approached significance for supportive, $F(2, 44) = 2.92$, $p = .06$, and ambivalent, $F(2, 35) = 2.63$, $p = .09$, friends. Subsequent analyses revealed that emotional support given by a purely positive friend was associated with smaller increases in CO reactivity when compared with those in the no-support group ($p < .01$) only. The opposite pattern, however, was found with ambivalent friends; that is, interacting with an ambivalent friend was associated with increases in CO reactivity when in the emotional support group compared to the no-support group ($p = .07$) only.

In addition, a significant Relationship Type × Type of Support interaction was found for TPR, $F(2, 74) = 3.81$, $p < .03$. As depicted in Figure 2 (bottom), analyses of the simple main effects for support type was near significant for ambivalent, $F(2, 35) = 2.95$, $p = .06$, but not supportive, $F(2, 44) = 1.12$, ns, friends. Specific contrasts of the differing support types within the ambivalent friend condition showed that emotional support was associated with smaller increases in TPR ($p < .09$) compared to the no-support condition only.[3]

DISCUSSION

This study was conducted to examine the contextual factors that could alter the effects of social support on cardiovascular reactivity in women. Consistent with our expectations, relationship quality was an important factor and moderated the influence of other social transactions on cardiovascular functioning. It is also important to point out that the manipulation checks provided strong evidence for the validity of our independent variables. The stressor was highly effective in increasing perceived stress and cardiovascular function, and individuals were clearly able to distinguish between the different types of support. Replicating prior research, women were also perceived as more emotionally supportive than men. Finally, supportive and ambivalent ties were comparable in their rated levels of positivity and differed only on the level of perceived negativity in the relationships.

One of the main conclusions of our study is that social relationships may have both stress- buffering and stress-enhancing effects on the cardiovascular system of women, depending on the quality of the relationship. For instance, we found that women interacting with ambivalent female friends had significantly higher levels of DBP, TPR, and PEP reactivity compared to women interacting with supportive female friends. These findings are interpretable in light of prior research on friendship processes in women. Male–female friendships have been

---

[3]The only effect that did not involve relationship type was a Gender of Friend × Support Type interaction for pre-ejection period (PEP) reactivity, $F(2, 74) = 3.19$, $p < .05$. Follow-up contrasts suggest that instrumental support provided by male friends was associated with a shortening of PEP (indicating greater sympathetic control of the heart) compared to the emotional support condition only ($p < .05$).

described in the literature as less intimate and less stable (Davis & Todd, 1985) than female–female friendships. Opposite-sex friends are also less likely to interact with one another (Rands & Levinger, 1979) and to share similar interests. These differences imply that women are more likely to be sensitive to the reactions of a female friend. As a result, women interacting with ambivalent, female friends may feel the most threatened and evaluated because the feedback offered could be interpreted in a more negative light. Consistent with this explanation, women accompanied by a female, ambivalent friend rated the task to be harder and viewed them as more dominant than participants in the other conditions.

The moderation of cardiovascular reactivity via relationship quality was also evident on CO and TPR reactivity. For instance, receiving emotional support from a purely positive friend was related to smaller increases in CO compared to the no-support condition. Therefore, emotional supportive messages may be helpful because they convey the initial expressions of care, concern, affection, and understanding of a person's distress and it occurs in the context of a primarily positive relationship (Burleson & Goldsmith, 1998). Instrumental support, in contrast, may be less effective because the emotional support derived from those messages is less direct. In retrospect, it is also possible that instrumental support did not reduce reactivity because it may carry an additional evaluative component, implying the person is not as capable of handling the task (Bolger, Zuckerman, & Kessler, 2000).

In contrast, receiving emotional support from an ambivalent friend was related to increases in CO and smaller increases in TPR when compared to individuals in the no-support condition. This pattern of effects was unexpected and hence difficult to explain. If replicable, future research using measures of specific task appraisals may help clarify the processes potentially underlying these results (Tomaka, Blascovich, Kibler, & Ernst, 1997).

It is important to point out that we did not replicate prior research on the beneficial influence of provided support as we found no main effect of support type on cardiovascular reactivity. It is difficult to compare our study with prior research because we used a more indirect method of manipulating social support to decrease the potential evaluation associated with the friend. However, in retrospect, it may be possible that the cardiovascular effects associated with this manipulation were weaker than prior research because the friend was not actually present providing the support. Future research that directly compares such experimental conditions would help to clarify this issue.

When considered collectively, there are some important implications of these results that also suggest directions for future study. First and perhaps most important, the results highlight the usefulness of considering both positivity and negativity in the context of women's close relationships. We would again like to emphasize that most prior research on social support typically only assesses the level of positivity in relationships. However, this procedure would miss the heterogeneity that exists within important social ties and would have obscured the different reactivity effects we found for ambivalent and supportive friends.

The potential daily life correlates of our laboratory study with ambivalent and supportive ties are also worth discussing. Despite the reactivity differences found in this study, one might argue that in real life individuals can avoid ambivalent relationships and hence these relationships are less consequential. To investigate this possibility, we conducted ancillary analyses in which we examined whether ambivalent and supportive ties differed on rated relationship contact and importance. Results revealed that supportive and ambivalent friends were not rated as significantly different on either of these variables. Thus, there appears to be ample opportunity for interactions with ambivalent ties to influence cardiovascular function in everyday life. Further, in a recent study we found that interactions with individuals one felt ambivalent toward were associated with higher levels of ambulatory SBP during daily life compared to interactions with supportive, indifferent, or more purely negative ties (Holt-Lunstad, Uchino, & Smith, 2000).

This study also suggests that specific psychological processes may underlie how and when support is effective in reducing reactivity. As such, future studies might also benefit from assessments based on the interpersonal circumplex as it was informative in providing converging evidence for some of our physiological findings. The more widespread use of the interpersonal circumplex should prove useful in social psychophysiological studies as they (a) are well- validated, (b) appear sensitive to variations in the social context, and (c) allow for meaningful comparisons across studies (Smith et al., 1998; Smith et al., in press).

There are several limitations of this study that need to be discussed. First, this study was constructed to test how individuals would react physiologically to the receipt of social support. It is often the case that individuals first make decisions about whether they should seek social support. Because the effect of receiving support may be different when a person actively seeks support versus when it is simply given, caution needs to be taken when interpreting these findings to all possible social support transactions. In addition, although we found several significant interactions with relationship quality, this study may have been underpowered to examine the higher order statistical interactions or statistical interactions characterized by smaller effect sizes. For instance, power estimates in this study indicate that we only had adequate power for detecting a moderate to large effect size (Cohen, J.,1988).

It is also important to point out that participants selected their friends to accompany them to this study. As a result, there may be some underlying personality differences that influenced the section process and thus may be driving some of these effects. For instance, individuals high in trait hostility tend to have lower levels of social support (Smith, 1992). In this study, individual differences in trait hostility were not significantly related to bringing in supportive or ambivalent friends ($F < 1.17$). In our prior research, we have also not found the number of ambivalent network members to be associated with trait negative affect or hostility levels (Uchino et al., 2001). Nevertheless, more research is needed on the personality correlates of social networks and its potential to clarify links between social relationships and health outcomes.

A final limitation of the study concerns the generalizability of the study sample. This study only included female, college-aged participants who were healthy. The extent to which these findings can be expanded to people of different age groups, ethnic groups, or health status cannot be known. Similarly, research designs should also be carried out that include men in the sample. Men's friendships with other men and women are characteristically different from women's friendships and this may have important implications for this study. For instance, men may appraise the receipt of support from their friends differently from women and may actually benefit more from instrumental support (Winstead, Derlega, Lewis, Sanchez-Hucles, & Clarke, 1992). It was not logistically possible in this study to include both women and men as participants as it would have significantly increased our already large sample size using time-intensive methods (i.e., impedance cardiography data collection and reduction). Of course, this limitation does not invalidate the results generated by this study because women are generally underrepresented in behavioral medicine research. In fact, this study points to some of the interpersonal processes that may result in stress-buffering or stress-enhancing effects of close relationships for women.

REFERENCES

Allen, K. M., Blascovich, J., Tomaka, J., & Kelsey, R. M. (1991). Presence of human friends and pet dogs as moderators of autonomic responses to stress in women. *Journal of Personality and Social Psychology, 61,* 582–589.

Barbee, A. P., Gulley, M. R., & Cunningham, M. R. (1990). Support seeking in personal relationships. *Journal of Social and Personal Relationships, 7,* 531–540.

Barrera, M. (1980). A method of assessment of social support networks in community survey research. *Connections, 3,* 8–13.

Berkman, L. F. (1995). The role of social relations in health promotion. *Psychosomatic Medicine, 57,* 245–254.

Berntson, G. G., Quigley, K. S., Jang, J., & Boysen, S. (1990). An approach to artifact identification: Application to heart period data. *Psychophysiology, 27,* 586–598.

Bolger, N., Zuckerman, A., & Kessler, R. C. (2000). Invisible support and adjustment to stress. *Journal of Personality and Social Psychology, 79,* 953–961.

Burke, R. J., & Weir, T. (1978). Sex differences in adolescent life stress, social support, and well-being. *Journal of Psychology, 98,* 277–288.

Burleson, B. R., & Goldsmith, D. J. (1998). How the comforting process works: Alleviating emotional distress through conversationally induced reappraisals. In P. A. Andersen & L. K. Guerrero (Eds.), *Handbook of communication and emotion: Research, theory, applications, and contexts* (pp. 245–280). San Diego, CA: Academic.

Christenfeld, N., Gerin, W., Wolfgang, L., Sanders, M., et al. (1997). Social support effects on cardiovascular reactivity: Is a stranger as effective as a friend? *Psychosomatic Medicine, 59,* 388–398.

Cohen, J. (1988). *Statistical power analyses for the behavioral sciences.* Hillsdale, NJ: Lawrence Erlbaum Associates, Inc.

Cohen, S. (1988). Psychosocial models of the role of social support in the etiology of physical disease. *Health Psychology, 7,* 269–297.

Cohen, S., & Wills, T. A. (1985). Stress, social support, and the buffering hypothesis. *Psychological Bulletin, 98,* 310–357.

Coyne, J. C., & DeLongis, A. (1986). Going beyond social support: The role of social relationships in adaptation. *Journal of Consulting and Clinical Psychology, 54,* 454–460.

Davis, K. E., & Todd, M. J. (1985). Assessing friendship: Prototypes, paradigm cases, and relationship description. In S. W. Duck & D. Perlman (Eds.), *Understanding personal relationships: An interdisciplinary approach* (pp. 17–28). Newbury Park, CA: Sage.

Fincham, F. D., & Linfield, K. J. (1997). A new look at marital quality: Can spouses feel positive and negative about their marriages? *Journal of Family Psychology, 11,* 489–502.

Flaherty, J., & Richman, J. (1989). Gender differences in the perception and utilization of social support: Theoretical perspectives and an empirical test. *Social Science and Medicine, 28,* 1221–1228.

Fiore, J., Becker, J., & Coppel, D. B. (1983). Social network interactions: A buffer or a stress? *American Journal of Community Psychology, 11,* 423–439.

Glynn, L. A., Christenfeld, N., & Gerin, W. (1999). Gender, social support, and cardiovascular responses to stress. *Psychosomatic Medicine, 61,* 234–242.

Holt-Lunstad, J., Uchino, B. N., & Smith, T. W. (2000). Relationship quality predicts ambulatory blood pressure during social interactions. *Psychophysiology, 37,* S49.

House, J. S., Landis, K. R., & Umberson, D. (1988). Social relationships and health. *Science, 241,* 540–545.

Jennings, J. R., Kamarck, T., Stewart, C., Eddy, M., & Johnson, P. (1992). Alternate cardiovascular baseline assessment techniques: Vanilla or resting baseline. *Psychophysiology, 24,* 474–475.

Kamarck, T. W., Jennings, J. R., Debski, T. T., Glickman-Weiss, E., Johnson, P. S., Eddy, M. J., & Manuck, S. B. (1992). Reliable measures of behaviorally evoked cardiovascular reactivity form a PC-based test battery: Results from student and community samples. *Psychophysiology, 29,* 17–28.

Kiecolt-Glaser, J. K., Dura, J. R., Speicher, C. E., Trask, J. O., & Glaser, R. (1991). Spousal caregivers of dementia victims: Longitudinal changes in immunity and health. *Psychosomatic Medicine, 53,* 345–362.

Kiecolt-Glaser, K. G., & Newton, T. L. (2001). Marriage and health: His and hers. *Psychological Bulletin, 127,* 472–503.

Kiesler, D. J. (1991). Interpersonal methods of assessment and diagnosis. In C. R. Snyder & D. R. Forsyth (Eds.), *Handbook of social and clinical psychology: The health perspective.* Elmsford, NY: Pergamon.

Lepore, S. J. (1998). Problems and prospects for the social support-reactivity hypothesis. *Annals of Behavioral Medicine, 20,* 257–269.

Lepore, S. J., Allen, K. A. M., & Evans, G. W. (1993). Social support lowers cardiovascular reactivity to an acute stressor. *Psychosomatic Medicine, 55,* 518–524.

Llabre, M. M., Spitzer, S. B., Saab, P. G., Ironson, G. H., & Schneiderman, N. (1991). The reliability and specificity of delta versus residualized change as measures of cardiovascular reactivity to behavioral challenges. *Psychophysiology, 28,* 701–711.

Manuck, S. B. (1994). Cardiovascular reactivity in cardiovascular disease: "Once more unto the breach." *International Journal of Behavioral Medicine, 1,* 4–31.

Nuevo, Y., Cheng-Yu, D., & Mitra, S. (1984). Interpolated finite impulse response filters. *IEEE Transactions on Acoustics, Speech, and Signal processing, ASSP–32,* 563–570.

Rands, M., & Levinger, G. (1979). Implicit theories of relationship: An intergenerational study. *Journal of Personality and Social Psychology, 37,* 645–661.

Rook, K. S. (1984). The negative side of social interaction: Impact on psychological well being. *Journal of Personality and Social Psychology, 72,* 1349–1363.

Seeman, T. E. (1996). Social ties and health: The benefits of social integration. *Annals of Epidemiology, 6,* 442–451.

Sherwood, A., Allen, M., Fahrenberg, J., Kelsey, R., Lovallo, W., & Van Doorman, L. (1990). Methodological guidelines for impedence cardiography. *Psychophysiology, 27,* 1–23.

Shumaker, S. A., & Hill, D. R. (1991). Gender differences in social support and health. *Health Psychology, 10,* 102–111.

Smith, T. W. (1992). Hostility and health: Current status of a psychosomatic hypothesis. *Health Psychology, 11,* 139–150.

Smith, T. W., Gallo, L. C., Goble, L., Ngu, L. Q., & Stark, K. A. (1998). Agency, communion, and cardiovascular reactivity during marital interaction. *Health Psychology, 17,* 537–545.

Smith, T. W., Gallo, L. C., & Ruiz, J. M. (in press). Towards a social psychophysiology of cardiovascular reactivity: Interpersonal concepts and methods in the study of stress and coronary disease. In J. Suls & K. Wallston (Eds.), *Social psychological foundations of health and illness.* Oxford, England: Blackwell.

Smith, T. W., Limon, J. P., Gallo, L. C., & Ngu, L. Q. (1996). Interpersonal control and cardiovascular reactivity: Goals, behavioral expression, and the moderating effects of sex. *Journal of Personality and Social Psychology, 70,* 1012–1024.

Smith, T. W., Nealey, J. B., Kircher, J. C., & Limon, J. P. (1997). Social determinants of cardiovascular reactivity: Effects of incentive to exert influence and evaluative threat. *Psychophysiology, 34,* 65–73.

Tomaka, J., Blascovich, J., Kibler, J., & Ernst, J. M. (1997). Cognitive and physiological antecedents of threat and challenge appraisal. *Journal of Personality and Social Psychology, 73,* 63–72.

Trobst, K. K. (2000). An interpersonal conceptualization and quantification of social support transactions. *Personality and Social Psychology Bulletin, 26,* 971–986.

Uchino, B. N., Cacioppo, J. T., & Kiecolt-Glaser, J. K. (1996). The relationship between social support and physiological processes: A review with emphasis on underlying mechanisms and implications for health. *Psychological Bulletin, 119,* 488–531.

Uchino, B. N., Holt-Lunstad, J., Uno, D., & Flinders, J. B. (2001). Heterogeneity in the social networks of young and older adults: Prediction of mental health and cardiovascular reactivity during acute stress. *Journal of Behavioral Medicine, 24,* 361–382.

Umberson, D. (1987). Family status and health behaviors: Social control as a dimension of social integration. *Journal of Health and Social Behavior, 28,* 306–319.

Winstead, B. A., Derlega, V. J., Lewis, R. J., Sanchez-Hucles, J., & Clarke, E. (1992). Friendship, social interaction, and coping with stress. *Communication Research, 19,* 193–211.

Wiggins, J. S., & Broughton, R. (1991). A geometric taxonomy of personality scales. *European Journal of Personality, 5,* 343–365.

Wiggins, J. S., Trapnell, P., & Phillips, N. (1988). Psychometric and geometric characteristics of the revised Interpersonal Adjective Scales (IAS–B5). *Multivariate Behavioral Research, 23,* 517–530.

INTERNATIONAL JOURNAL OF BEHAVIORAL MEDICINE, 9(3), 263–285
Copyright © 2002, Lawrence Erlbaum Associates, Inc.

Which Aspects of Socio-Economic Status are Related to Health in Mid-Aged and Older Women?

Gita D. Mishra, Kylie Ball, Annette J. Dobson, Julie E. Byles, and Penny Warner-Smith

A population-based study was conducted to validate gender- and age-specific indexes of socio-economic status (SES) and to investigate the associations between these indexes and a range of health outcomes in 2 age cohorts of women. Data from 11,637 women aged 45 to 50 and 9,510 women aged 70 to 75 were analyzed. Confirmatory factor analysis produced four domains of SES among the mid-aged cohort (employment, family unit, education, and migration) and four domains among the older cohort (family unit, income, education, and migration). Overall, the results supported the factor structures derived from another population-based study (Australian Bureau of Statistics, 1995), reinforcing the argument that SES domains differ across age groups. In general, the findings also supported the hypotheses that women with low SES would have poorer health outcomes than higher SES women, and that the magnitude of these effects would differ according to the specific SES domain and by age group, with fewer and smaller differences observed among older women. The main excep-

Kylie Ball, School of Health Sciences, Deakin University, Victoria, Australia; Annette J. Dobson, School of Population Health, University of Queensland, Queensland, Australia; Julie E. Byles, Centre for Clinical Epidemiology & Biostatistics, University of Newcastle, Australia; Penny Warner-Smith, Department of Leisure and Tourism Studies, University of Newcastle, Australia.

The research on which this article is based was conducted as part of the Australian Longitudinal Study on Women's Health (Women's Health Australia).

Kylie Ball is supported by a Public Health Postdoctoral Research Fellowship from the Australian National Health and Medical Research Council, ID 136925.

We are grateful to the Australian Commonwealth Department of Health and Ageing for funding and to the staff of the Research Centre for Gender and Health at the University of Newcastle, Australia, for their assistance. We are also grateful to the editor and referees for their helpful comments and suggestions.

Correspondence concerning this article should be addressed to Kylie Ball, School of Health Sciences, Deakin University, 221 Burwood Highway, Burwood VIC 3125, Australia. E-mail: kball@deakin.edu.au

tion was that in the older cohort, the education domain was significantly associated with specific health conditions. Results suggest that relations between SES and health are highly complex and vary by age, SES domain, and the health outcome under study.

Key words: socio-economic status (SES), measurement, physical and mental health, health care utilization, health behavior, women's health

A vast body of research demonstrates associations between socio-economic status (SES) and morbidity and mortality from a range of physical and mental health conditions. Low SES has been linked with the prevalence of cardiovascular disease (Brezinka & Kittel, 1996; Hallqvist, Lundbert, Diderichsen, & Ahlbom, 1998; McElduff & Dobson, 2000; Osler et al., 2000; Tyroler, 1999), obesity (Sarlio-Lahteenkorva & Lahelma, 1999; Sobal & Stunkard, 1989), Type 2 diabetes (Evans, Newton, Ruta, MacDonald, & Morris, 2000), hypertension (Vargas, Ingram, & Gillum, 2000), complaints and symptoms (Der, MacIntyre, Ford, Hunt, & West, 1999; Mackenbach, 1992), including constipation (Johanson & Sonnenberg, 1990), perceived general health (Hemingway, Nicholson, Stafford, Roberts, & Marmot, 1997; Mackenbach, 1992), and psychosocial stress (Mackenbach, 1992). Those with low SES are also reportedly at increased risk of engaging in unhealthy behaviors including smoking (Graham & Hunt, 1994; Power & Matthews, 1997), poor diet (Baghurst et al., 1990), physical inactivity (Crespo, Ainsworth, Keteyian, Heath, & Smit, 1999), and decreased use of health care services (Mackenbach, 1992).

SES inequalities in health may vary by gender and age. There is some inconsistency in results of studies that have compared SES differentials among men and women. Although some findings demonstrate stronger associations of SES with health outcomes among men (e.g., Arber, 1997; Elo & Preston, 1996), others show no sex differences (e.g., Hemingway et al., 1997). Some evidence suggests that inequalities increase over the adult years until later in life (House et al., 1994) and that SES differences in relative rates of mortality and morbidity are strongest among young to mid-aged adults (Mustard, Derksen, Bethelot, Wolfson, & Roos, 1997). It has been suggested that SES inequalities in health and mortality are small in the elderly, perhaps due to a narrowing of social and economic differentials once individuals leave employment (Anderson, Sorlie, Backlund, Johnson, & Kaplan, 1997). However, these findings may depend on country- or time-specific findings, such as social welfare support for the elderly. In addition, contradictory findings show SES gradients in health do exist among the elderly (Berkman & Gurland, 1998; Broom, 1984; Hart, Davey Smith, & Blane, 1998). Studies showing a narrowing of SES differentials among older adults have tended to rely on income as an indicator of SES, and the inclusion of education in addition to income in the study by Berkman and Gurland (1998) may have contributed to its contradictory findings.

Such contradictory findings and use of varying indicators is likely to be attributable in part to disagreement over the conceptualization of SES. SES is the term commonly used to refer to the expression and distribution of such attributes as occupation, income, and status (Liberatos, Link, & Kelsey, 1988), although Kreiger et al. (1997) preferred the term *socio-economic position*, arguing that SES includes both access to and possession of material resources as well as prestige and position in a hierarchical ranking. According to seminal researcher Max Weber, differential social position is based on three dimensions: class (an economic concept, indicated, e.g., by income), power (related to political context), and status ("access to life chances" based on social and cultural factors; Liberatos et al., 1988; Weber, 1946). According to this definition, factors such as family background and lifestyle could be considered sociocultural factors reflective of the "status" dimension (Liberatos et al., 1988). Although not typically considered a component of SES, it is also now recognized that "ethnicity" is a social rather than biological construct (Kreiger, 2000) and ethnicity and migration history may also reflect "access to life chances." Migrants in Australia, for example, experience higher rates of unemployment and lower labor force participation rates than the Australian-born population (Australian Bureau of Statistics [ABS], 1999). This may be attributable to noneconomic factors, including migrants' experiences of discrimination in their new country. Although associations between health and SES are commonly explained in terms of the material reality of modern life, it is important to acknowledge the complex contribution of social, cultural, and behavioral factors (Scambler & Higgs, 1999), particularly when considering mental, as well as physical, health. Structural disadvantage and poorer life chances shape psychosocial orientations and lifestyle behaviors that are prejudicial to health. Hence the inclusion of migrant history as a social indicator along with conventional measures of SES provides a broader picture of socio-economic position and its association with a range of physical and mental health outcomes. Although we accept the "blurring" of material and social power that occurs with the use of SES, we adopt SES rather than *socio-economic position* in this article as the more widely understood term.

The measurement of SES is particularly problematic for women, because previously typically used methods of assigning SES, such as allocating a woman the occupational class of her husband, are often inappropriate (Koskinen & Martelin, 1994; McDonough, Williams, House, & Duncan, 1999). The increasing labor force participation rate of women, which is seeing dual earning as the most common form of family life (Bradley, 1998), now affords the potential to analyze patterns of inequalities in health using women's own occupational status, and in fact demands that this be done (Arber, 1997; Baxter, 1991). Similarly, measures such as income or occupation are often not appropriate for assigning SES to older adults, who may be retired and/or on pensions (Daniel, 1984). The applicability of the SES measures to the specific populations being studied is critical (Liberatos et al., 1988). With older adults in particular, most research has used only limited indicators (notably education or income). In one of the few studies to investigate the use of multiple indexes of SES among older adults (Robert & House, 1996), it was found that the association between financial assets and health remained until quite late in life, and financial assets become a more important predictor of some measures of health than either education or income. This finding lends strength to claims that relying on a single indicator of SES is problematic, because different indicators of SES have different associations with specific health outcomes (e.g., Chandola, 2000). The use of several indicators, or of multidimensional methods of assigning SES, has been recommended (Liberatos et al., 1988; Martikainen, 1995).

In a recent study that attempted to address these problems, a set of individual-based, age-, and gender-specific indexes for assigning SES was developed (Mishra, Ball, Dobson, Byles, & Warner-Smith, 2001). Factor analysis of data from the 1995 Australian National Health Survey (NHS; ABS, 1995) produced consistent results that were interpreted in terms of five conceptually meaningful domains or factors of SES: employment, income, migration, family unit, and education. A factor can be interpreted as a dimension or construct that is a condensed statement of the relations between a set of variables (Kline, 1994). Results showed that age- and gender-specific SES scores based on these factors had stronger associations with physical and mental health than either an area-based index or the SES indicators developed in this study for middle-aged (40- to 44-year-old) men, and applied to the other age and gender groups. These results were interpreted as evidence that SES measures composed of social and demographic items demonstrate important age- and gender-specific differences that are relevant for health. However, further validation of the SES indexes, and investigation of their predictive ability for a range of health outcomes, is required.

The baseline surveys for the Australian Longitudinal Study on Women's Health (also known as the Women's Health Australia [WHA] project) presented an opportunity to examine these issues as they relate to women. Four main hypotheses examined in this article are:

1. The age-specific SES domains (employment, family unit, income, migration, and education) for women obtained for the NHS data will be replicated in the WHA data.

2. Self-reported measures of health will differ among SES groups defined for each of the SES domains, with women in low SES reporting poorer health outcomes than higher SES women.

3. The magnitude of SES differentials will vary among SES domains for different aspects of health; specifically, it is hypothesized that physical health and health care utilization will show stronger associations with economic domains and mental health will show stronger associations with sociocultural domains.

4. The SES differentials in health measures will be smaller for the older cohort than for the mid-aged cohort.

METHOD

The WHA project is a longitudinal study of factors affecting the health and well-being of three national cohorts of women who were aged 18 to 23 years ("young"), 45 to 50 years ("mid-aged"), and 70 to 75 years ("older") at the time of Survey 1 in 1996. This study, which is designed to track the health of women over a period of up to 20 years, will provide longitudinal data on health, health service use, sociodemographics, and personal information from 41,500 women. Since Survey 1, the three age cohorts have been surveyed annually on a rolling basis. It was not feasible to include the young cohort in this study, because education is known to be an important indicator of SES, and many of the young cohort of women were still in the process of acquiring educational qualifications.

Study Sample

The original WHA study sample was selected randomly from the national Medicare health insurance database (which incorporates all residents of Australia regardless of age, including immigrants and refugees). Women from rural and remote areas of Australia are overrepresented in the sample. Further details of the recruitment methods have been described elsewhere (Brown et al., 1998).

At Survey 1, in 1996, a total of 14,065 mid-aged women and 12,624 older women responded to the mailed surveys. The mid age cohort was surveyed for the second time in 1998, and the older cohort in 1999. There were two versions of Survey 2—a long version administered via mail (mid- aged: $N = 11,637$; older: $N = 9,510$) and a short version consisting of only selected questions, which was administered via telephone interview (mid-aged: $N = 691$; older: $N = 920$). The response rates for Survey 2 were 92% (for the mid-aged) and 91% (for older women) of those women who had consented at Survey 1 to further contact and had not subsequently died. The nonrespondents consisted of those who did not return Survey 2 (mid-aged: 6.5%; older: 7.6%) and those who declined to participate (mid-aged: 1.5%; and older: 1.8%). Women who responded to the short version of Survey 2 were excluded from the analyses because some of the variables relevant to this article were not collected in the short version of the survey. The sample for this study consisted of the 11,637 mid-aged women and 9,510 older women who responded to both surveys.

Measures

All of the demographic and socio-economic items in Surveys 1 and 2 were selected for analysis (25 items for the mid-aged women and 18 items for older women). For a few items, some categories have been collapsed due to small numbers of women. Most of the demographic and socio-economic items used in the analyses were collected in Survey 1. The items selected, and their response options, are outlined in Table 1.

A range of health conditions and behaviors that have been established in previous studies to be associated with indicators of SES were selected from Survey 1 as indicators of health.

1. Health conditions: Three specific health conditions that are known to be associated with SES were selected for inclusion in analyses. These conditions were: having ever been told by a doctor they had hypertension (two response options), being told by a doctor they had diabetes (two response options), and experiencing constipation in the last 12 months (four response options from *never* to *often*; responses of *sometimes* and *often* were used to estimate the prevalence).

2. Medical Outcomes Study Health Survey Short-Form (SF–36): Participants completed the SF–36 (Ware, Kosinski, & Keller, 1994), a widely used and validated measure of health-related quality of life, separated into physical and mental health component summary scores denoted as physical health (PCS) and mental health (MCS), respectively.

3. Health care utilization: The use of general practitioner services has been shown to be inversely related to SES levels (Young, Dobson & Byles, 2001). To measure the number of times health services were utilized in the last 12 months, respondents were asked, How many times have you consulted the following for *your own health* in the *last 12 months*? ... Family doctor or another general practitioner; hospital doctor; specialist doctor, allied health professional; "alternative" health practitioner. The response options were: none, once or twice, three or four times, five or six times, seven or more times. Responses were scored based on approximate annual frequencies of health care utilization (*none* = 0; *once or twice* = 1.5; *three or four times* = 3.5; *five or six times* = 5.5; *seven or more times* = 8). These were summed over the five different types of providers of health services to give an overall measure of health care utilization ranging from 0 to 40.

TABLE 1

Items and Response Options for the Items Included in Factor Analyses

Item	Order of Response Options (Number of Options)
Marital status	Never married/separated/divorced/widowed, married/defacto (2)
Country of birth	Other, Asia, Europe (Non-English speaking), Other English speaking, Australia (5)
Year of arrival in Australia	Mid cohort: 1966 or later,1965 or earlier, Australian born (3) Older cohort: 1956 or later,1955 or earlier, Australian born (3)
Usual language spoken at home	Non-English, English (2)
Area of residence	Other rural/remote areas, large/small rural centres, capital city/other metropolitan centres (3)
Employment status	Mid cohort only: No paid work (unemployed , studying, unpaid voluntary work, sick, other), home duties, work without pay (eg family business), Employed ûpart time, employed ûfull time (5)
Usual hours worked each week	Not applicable, 1û24, 25û40, 41 or more hours (4)
Whether in paid shift work	Not applicable, yes, no (3)
Whether in paid work at night	Not applicable, yes, no (3)
Occupation	Never had a paid job/other, manual workers/machine operators or drivers, sales and personal service workers/clerks, tradespersons/para-professional; professionals/managers or administrators (5)
Partner's occupation	Not applicable/never had a paid job/other, manual workers/machine operators or drivers, Sales and personal service workers/clerks, tradespersons/para-professional, professionals/managers or administrators (5)
Source of income for self/partner	
Wage or salary	Mid cohort: not applicable, no, yes (3)
Business/farm/partnership	Mid cohort: not applicable, no, yes (3)
Government pension or allowance	Older cohort: not applicable, no, yes
Superannuation or other private income	Older cohort: not applicable, no, yes
Gross personal income per annum	Mid cohort: Not applicable/don't know/not stated, $15,999 or less, $16,000–36,999, $37,000 or more (4)
Gross personal income of partner per annum	Mid cohort: not applicable/don't know/not stated, $15,999 or less, $16,000–36,999, $37,000 or more (4)
Highest qualification	Mid cohort: No formal qualification, School certificate, Higher school certificate, trade/apprenticeship/certificate/diploma, bachelor degree/higher degree (5) Older cohort: No formal qualification/School certificate, higher school certificate, Trade/apprenticeship/certificate/diploma/bachelor degree/higher degree (3)

(CONTINUED)

TABLE 1
(CONTINUED)

Item	Order of Response Options (Numger of Options)
Age first left school	Mid cohort: not applicable/16 years or younger, 17 years or older (2)
	Older cohort: Not applicable/14 years or younger, 15–16 years, 17 years or older (3)
Self reported class	Mid cohort: don't know/missing, working, middle/upper (3)
Whether has private hospital insurance coverage	No, Yes (2)
Whether has private health insurance for ancillary services	No, Yes (2)
Type of dwelling	Caravan/tent/cabin/houseboat/other, Flat/unit/apartment, house (3)
Name in the ownership/ purchasing/tenancy agreement	Not applicable/other family member/other, partner or spouse, self with partner or spouse, or self with others, or just self (3)
Whether lived alone	Yes, No (2)
Whether lived with partner or spouse	No, Yes (2)
Whether lived with own children	No, Yes (2)

4.   Height and weights: Self-reported height and weight were used to compute body mass index (BMI = weight in kilograms/square of height in meters). BMI was classified according to the Australian National Health and Medical Research Council (1997) guidelines: underweight (<20.00 kg/m²), acceptable weight (20.00-25.00 kg/m²), overweight (25.01–30.00kg/m²), and obese (>30.00kg/m².

5.   Health behaviors: Physical activity scores were derived from self-reported frequency and intensity of leisure time physical activity. Scores were classified as: none or low, moderate, or high level of physical activity (Brown, Mishra, Lee, & Bauman, 2000). Cigarette smoking status was defined as nonsmoker or smoker.

Statistical Analysis

All demographic and socio-economic items were considered as ordinal variables. For each item, response options were arranged in ascending order with respect to SES. A separate category was created for the response "not applicable." The order of the categories in each item are given in Table 1. With the sample stratified by age, confirmatory factor analysis using the method of principal components and varimax rotation was performed on the demographic and socio-economic items. Items that cross-loaded on several factors or had loadings of 0.5 or less on all the factors were subsequently eliminated. Inter-item reliability for each factor was assessed by Cronbach's coefficients for standardized variables. Kaiser's measure of sampling adequacy was used to quantify the degree of intercorrelation among the items and the appropriateness of factor analysis was also reported (Hair, Anderson, Tatham, & Black, 1997). In addition, the factor structures were compared with the results from the samples after they had been randomly split into two subsamples and the analyses repeated on each half.

Factor scores for each of the resultant SES domains were grouped into tertiles (or in some cases dichotomized). Univariate analyses (χ^2 test) and the Cochran–Armitage test for trend were used to compare percentages of women reporting medical history, symptoms, and health behaviors by SES tertiles (low, middle, and high SES). Multiple linear regression models were used to analyze the relation between physical health (the outcome variable) and the four SES domains simultaneously (four explanatory variables). The analyses were repeated for the outcome variables of mental health and health care utilization. Means and 95% confidence intervals (CI) were estimated for physical health, mental health, and health care utilization variables using the least square means option of the general linear models procedure of SAS (SAS Institute Inc., 1989). Bonferroni corrections were used to reduce the effects of inflated Type 1 errors due to multiple comparisons (Neter, Kutner, Nachtsheim, & Wasserman, 1996). To estimate the magnitude of SES differentials, mean difference and 95% confidence interval between the high and low tertiles were also calculated using means option of the general linear models procedure.

RESULTS

Factor analysis confirmed four independent factors for the mid-aged cohort and four independent factors for the older cohort. Table 2 sets out the factors, which together explain 66% and 69% of the variation in the data for the mid-aged and older women, respectively. The main difference was that the employment domain was the primary factor for the mid group; in the older group, this was replaced by the family unit domain followed by the income domain, which consisted of items relating to health insurance and source of income. The education and migration domains were the next most important factors for both cohorts.

Tables 3 and 4 show the relation between the SES domains and various health outcomes for the mid-aged cohort. Because the distribution of factor scores for the employment domain was bimodal, factor scores were dichotomized to low and high groups. For other factors, tertiles of scores were used, with the lowest tertile representing the most disadvantaged group. Physical and mental health scores generally increased across increasing SES tertiles,

TABLE 2
Items and Factor Loadings[a,f] Determining Socio-Economic Status Dimensions for Mid-Aged and Older Women

	Mid-Aged Women 45–50 (n = 11,637)				Older Women 70–75 (n = 9,510)			
Item	Factor 1 Employment	Factor 2 Family Unit	Factor 3 Education	Factor 4 Migration	Factor 1 Family Unit	Factor 2 Income	Factor 3 Education	Factor 4 Migration
Whether in paid work at night[b]	0.94							
Whether in paid shift work[b]	0.94							
Employment status	0.91							
Usual hours worked each week	0.86							
Source of income for self/partner – wage or salary	0.54							
Whether lived with partner or spouse		0.93			0.96			
Marital status		0.91			0.93			
Whether lived alone		0.72			0.93			
Partner's occupation		0.65						
Gross personal income of partner per annum		0.57						
Highest qualification			0.77				0.84	
Age first left school			0.69				0.74	
Occupation			0.64				0.74	
Self reported class			0.55					
Year of arrival in Australia				0.65				0.81
Usual language spoken at home				0.56				0.85
Whether has private hospital insurance						0.80		
Whether has private health insurance for ancillary services						0.79		
Source of income for self/partner- government pension or allowance						0.68		
Source of income for self/partner super-annuation or other private income						0.64		
Eigenvalue (% of variance explained)	4.1 (26%)	3.0 (19%)	1.9 (12%)	1.4 (9%)	3.0 (25%)	2.4 (20%)	1.6 (13%)	1.3 (11%)

[a]Factor loadings are correlations of an item with a factor. [b]About 50% of all shift workers reported that they were in paid work at night.

TABLE 3

Means, Confidence Intervals (CI) and *p* Values for Physical and Mental Health and Health Care Utilization in Mid-Aged Women

Mid	Tertile	Employment			Family Unit			Education			Migration		
		M	95% CI	p	M	95% CI	p	M	95% CI	p	M	95% CI	p
Physical health				<0.001			<0.001			<0.001			0.4
	Low	48.3	47.9 – 48.7		49.7	49.3 – 50.0		49.4	49.1 – 49.7		49.8	49.4 – 50.1	
	Middle[a]				50.4	50.0 – 50.8		50.7	50.4 – 51.0		49.9	49.5 – 50.2	
	High	51.6	51.3 – 51.8		51.5	51.1 – 51.8		51.5	51.2 – 51.8		50.2	49.8 – 50.5	
Difference in physical health between high and low SES tertiles		3.3	2.9 – 3.6	<0.001	1.8	1.3 – 2.4	<0.001	2.1	1.5 – 2.6	<0.01	0.4	−0.9 – 1.7	0.04
Mental Health				<0.001			<0.001			0.006			0.6
	Low	50.3	50.0 – 50.7		49.5	49.2 – 49.9		50.1	49.7 – 50.5		50.6	50.3 – 50.9	
	Middle[a]				51.2	50.9 – 51.5		51.3	50.9 – 51.7		50.7	50.4 – 51.1	
	High	51.1	50.9 – 51.4		51.9	51.6 – 52.2		51.2	50.8 – 51.6		50.9	50.5 – 51.2	
Difference in mental health between high and low SES tertiles		0.8	0.4 – 1.2	<0.001	2.3	1.8 – 2.9	<0.001	1.1	0.6 – 1.7	<0.01	0.3	−0.2 – 0.8	0.9
Health care utilization				<0.001			<0.001			0.02			0.6
	Low	8.5	8.3 – 8.7		8.3	8.1 – 8.6		8.0	7.7 – 8.2		7.9	7.7 – 8.2	
	Middle[a]				7.7	7.5 – 8.0		7.7	7.5 – 7.9		7.9	7.6 – 8.1	
	High	7.6	7.4 – 7.7		7.6	7.3 – 7.8		8.0	7.2 – 8.2		**7.8**	7.6 – 8.1	
Difference in health care utilisation between high and low SES tertiles		−1.0	−1.2 – −0.7	<0.001	−0.7	−1.1 – −0.4	<0.001	0.0	−0.3 – 0.3	0.7	−0.1	−0.4 – 0.3	0.6

Note. SES = socio-economic status.

[a]Because the distribution of the factor scores corresponding to the Employment domain was bimodal, groups were dichotomized to low and high employment status.

TABLE 4

Percentages Reporting Health Conditions and Behaviors, by Tertiles[a] of Socio Economic Status (SES) Domains, in Mid-Aged Women, and Difference (With 95% Confidence Interval) Between Low and High Tertiles

		Employment[a]			Family Unit			
	N	Low	High	Difference (95% CI)	Low	Mid	High	Difference (95% CI)
Health Condition								
Diabetes	342	3.9	2.3**	-1.6 (-1.7, -1.5)	3.4	2.7	1.8[b]**	-1.6 (-1.7, -1.5)
Hypertension	2,558	24.0	19.8**	-4.2 (-4.3, -4.1)	22.1	21.8	17.9[b]**	-4.20 (-4.25, -4.15)
Constipation	3,170	28.0	24.8**	-3.20 (-3.24, -3.16)	26.3	25.6	23.6[b]***	-2.7 (-2.74, -2.66)
Health behavior								
Current cigarette smoker	2,024	17.3	16.9	-0.4 (-0.5, -0.3)	21.0	15.0	12.7[b]**	-8.3 (-8.4, -8.3)
Physical activity level (moderate/vigorous)	5,144	44.2	41.2**	3.0 (-3.04, -2.94)	41.7	42.4	43.7	2.0 (1.96, 2.04)
Obesity (% obese/very obese)	2,142	23.0	16.5**	-6.5 (-6.6, -6.4)	20.1	19.1	15.4[b]**	-4.7 (-4.8, -4.6)

(CONTINUED)

TABLE 4
(CONTINUED)

	Education			Migration			
	Low	Mid	High	Difference (95% CI)	Low	Mid	High	Difference (95% CI)
Health Condition								
Diabetes	4.0	2.1	1.8[b]**	−2.2 (−2.3, −2.1)	3.1	2.8	2.0[b]**	−1.1 (−1.2, −1.0)
Hypertension	23.7	20.2	18.0[b]**	−5.7 (−5.75, 5.65)	20.0	22.0	19.8*	−0.2 (−0.25,−0.15)
Constipation	28.5	26.1	20.9[b]**	−7.6 (−7.64, −7.56)	26.9	24.9	23.8[b]**	−3.1 (−3.14,−3.06)
Health behavior								
Current cigarette smoker	20.2	16.9	11.7[b]**	−8.5 (−8.6, −8.4)	17.5	17.1	14.2[b]**	−3.3 (−3.4,−3.2)
Physical activity level (moderate/vigorous)	39.6	43.9	44.2[b]**	4.6 (4.57, 4.63)	42.4	41.2	44.2*	1.8 (1.76,1.84)
Obesity(% obese/very obese)	22.2	18.7	13.7[b]**	−8.5 (−8.6,−8.4)	17.4	20.4	16.7**	−0.7 (−0.8,−0.6)

[a]Since the distribution of the factor scores corresponding to the Employment domain was bimodal, groups were dichotomised to low and high employment status. [b]Cochran–Armitage test for linear trend: $P < 0.01$.χ^2 test for associations between health conditions and tertiles of SES domains:*$0.01 < p < 0.05$. **$p < 0.01$.

whereas health care utilization decreased for all domains. The most marked change occurred between the lowest tertile and the other two. For specific health measures shown in Table 4, there were significant linear trends across SES tertiles for the employment, family unit, and education domains except for cigarette smoking status (statistically significant for family unit and education only) and physical activity level (significant for employment and education only). Physical health differentials and health service utilization were largest for the employment domain and mental health differentials were largest for the family unit domain. Health behaviors and conditions differed most for the education domain.

There were substantially different relations between SES domains and health measures for the older cohort shown in Tables 5, and 6, with fewer statistically significant differences and smaller absolute differences. The family unit domain did not exhibit any significant associations with physical or mental health. The income domain had significant associations with the tertiles for mental health and health care utilization. As for the mid-aged cohort, physical and mental health generally increased across the education domain tertiles. With few exceptions, the only evidence of linear trends with specific health measures was found in the education domain. These tended to decline across education domain tertiles (with exceptions being physical activity, which markedly increased, and cigarette smoking, which was not significantly associated). The income domain showed significant differentials for cigarette smoking and obesity.

DISCUSSION

Overall, the results from the confirmatory factor analysis supported the factor structures derived from the NHS analysis with the exception of the housing domain, which did not appear in the WHA cohorts. This could be due to the different questions on housing included in each study. Five SES domains were identified overall, with four age-specific domains overlapping but differing slightly between mid-aged and older women. Age differences were consistent with those found in NHS analyses (Mishra et al., 2001). As expected, employment was not the primary factor among the older cohort, as only a small proportion of that age group reported that they were still in paid employment. Other income items such as gross personal annual income rarely appeared in the factors. This may be due to the high level (approximately 20%) of "don't know," "don't want to answer," or missing responses.

The results also supported the second and third hypotheses; namely that the SES groups would differ on health outcomes and that the magnitude of these SES differentials would vary according to the SES domain and health measure examined. Consistent with a vast body of previous research, results provide evidence of an inverse relation between SES and self-reported health. This study advanced

TABLE 5
Means, Confidence Intervals (CI) and P Values for Physical and Mental Health and Health Care Utilization in Older Women

Tertiles	Family Unit M	95% CI	p	Income M	95% CI	p	Education M	95% CI	p	Migration[a] M	95% CI	p
Physical health			0.5			0.06			<0.001			0.6
Low	50.9	50.4–51.4		50.7	50.2–51.2		50.1	49.6–50.6		50.7	50.2–51.4	
Middle[a]	50.8	50.3–51.3		50.7	50.1–51.1		50.8	50.3–51.2				
High	50.8	50.3–51.3		51.2	50.7–51.7		51.5	51.0–52.0		50.5	50.5–51.1	
Difference in physical health between high and low SES tertiles	0.0	−0.6–0.7	1.0	0.5	−0.2–1.2	0.06	1.5	0.7–2.2	<0.001	0.05	−0.5–0.6	0.6
Mental Health			0.2			<0.001			<0.001			0.001
Low	51.4	50.6–51.5		51.0	50.6–51.4		50.2	49.7–50.7		50.5	50.0–51.2	
Middle[a]	51.5	50.4–51.3		51.0	50.8–51.4		51.8	51.3–52.3				
High	51.4	50.9–51.8		52.2	51.8–52.6		52.2	51.7–52.7		51.6	51.4–51.9	
Difference in mental health between high and low SES tertiles	0.0	−0.6–0.5	0.8	1.2	0.5–1.7	<0.001	2.0	1.3–2.7	<0.001	1.1	0.5–1.6	0.001
Health care utilization			0.01			<0.001			0.7			0.6
Low	10.0	9.6–10.3		9.2	8.9–9.5		9.9	9.6–10.3		9.6	9.3–10.0	
Middle[a]	10.1	9.8–10.5		9.7	9.5–10.0		9.7	9.4–10.0				
High	9.2	8.9–9.5		10.3	10.1–10.6		9.7	9.4–10.0		9.8	9.6–10.0	
Difference in health care utilization between high and low SES tertiles	−0.7	−1.1–−0.4	0.03	1.2	0.8–1.5	<0.001	−0.2	−0.7–−0.2	0.7	0.2	−0.2–−0.6	0.6

Note. SES = Socio-economic status.

[a]Because the distribution of the factor scores corresponding to the Migration domain was bimodal, groups were dichotomized to low and high migration status.

TABLE 6
Percentages Reporting Health Conditions and Behaviors, by Tertiles of Socio-Economic Status (SES) Domains, in Older Women, and Difference (With 95% Confidence Interval [CI]) Between Low and High Tertiles

	N	Family Unit				Income			
		Low	Mid	High	Difference (95% CI)	Low	Mid	High	Difference (95% CI)
Health Condition									
Diabetes	840	7.8	7.8	7.9	0.1 (0.0, 0.2)	8.8	8.0	6.8	-2.0 (-2.1, -1.9)
Hypertension	4915	48.2	47.8	47.6	-0.60 (-0.64, -0.56)	49.1	48.8	45.8	-3.30 (-3.34, -3.24)
Constipation	2607	27.5	25.3	22.2**	-5.3 (-5.4, -5.2)	25.4	26.3	23.3	-2.1 (-2.2, -2.0)
Health behaviors									
Current cigarette smoker	704	5.6	6.1	7.5*	1.9 (1.8, 2.0)	9.1	5.9	4.2**b	-4.9 (-5.0, -4.8)
Physical activity (% moderate/ vigorous)	4417	43.8	45.8	48.0*	4.20 (4.16, 4.24)	45.7	44.9	47.0	1.30 (1.26, 1.34)
Obesity (% obese / very obese)	1379	14.1	13.1	14.2	0.1 (0.0, 0.2)	15.4	14.7	11.3**b	-4.1 (-4.2, -4.0)

(CONTINUED)

TABLE 6
(CONTINUED)

	Education				Migration[a]		
	Low	Mid	High	Difference (95% CI)	Low	High	Difference (95% CI)
Health Condition							
Diabetes	10.2	7.2	6.2**b	-4.0	8.2	7.8	-0.4
				(-4.1, -3.9)			(-0.5, -0.3)
Hypertension	51.4	48.2	44.1**b	-7.3	45.0	48.7*	3.7
				(-7.34, -7.26)			(3.66, 3.74)
Comstipation	30.5	23.5	21.0**b	-9.5	26.4	24.6	-1.8
				(-9.6, -9.4)			(-1.9, -1.7)
Health Behaviors							
Current cigarette smoker	5.9	5.9	7.5	1.6	8.1	5.9**	-2.2
				(1.5, 1.7)			(-2.3, -2.1)
Physical activity (% moderate/vigorous)	39.5	44.5	53.6**b	14.10	47.6	45.4	-2.20
				(14.06, 14.14)			(-2.24, -2.16)
Obesity (% obese/ very obese)	16.7	13.7	11.0**b	-5.7	14.6	13.6	-1.0
				(-5.8, -5.6)			(-1.1, -0.9)

[a]Because the distribution of the factor scores corresponding to the "Migration" domain was bimodal, groups were dichotomised to low and high migration status. χ^2 test for associations between health conditions and tertiles of SES domains.
[b]Cochran–Armitage test for linear trend: $p < .01$. $*.01 < p < .05$. $**p < .01$.

279

previous findings by showing that the magnitude of the SES–health associations differed depending on SES domain and the specific health outcome, with mental health differentials larger for economic aspects of SES (e.g., employment), but physical health and health care utilization differentials larger for sociocultural aspects (e.g., family unit). The results also partly supported the final hypothesis that SES differentials in health measures would be smaller for the older cohort than for the mid-aged cohort. The main exception was that in the older cohort, education was significantly associated with all the specific health measures, except health care utilization. This may be attributable to the likelihood that education level is stable in later adult life, unlike family unit or income, which are affected by widowhood or ceasing employment. Hence older women may become a more homogenous group in terms of their family situation and income, whereas differentials in education and associations with health outcomes remain. However, certain aspects (e.g., mental health and health care utilization) were significantly associated with either income or family unit. The implications of these findings for future research into health inequalities are that different domains of SES may be useful for identifying aspects of SES that are important for different health outcomes, but that at a minimum, education should be included as a measure of the SES of older adults.

The migration domain was found to be associated with symptoms (diabetes, hypertension, constipation) and health behaviors but not with self-rated physical and mental health or health care utilization. This may reflect cultural differences in perceptions of health. Further research into discrepancies between perceived and objective health in migrant groups is warranted, because the findings have implications for the responsiveness of the health care system to the needs of migrant women.

The fact that the relations between most of the SES domains and health outcomes were significant and meaningful (in terms of size of effects) when included in the regression models simultaneously (particularly for mid-aged women) demonstrates that these SES domains are independent predictors of health outcomes. In conjunction with findings that the magnitude of SES–health associations differed according to SES domain, these results suggest that different domains of SES are independently associated with different health outcomes. Acknowledging this study's cross-sectional design, these findings may reflect different pathways through which aspects of SES impact on health.

The findings support the validity of the measures developed in an earlier study by Mishra et al. (2001), reinforcing the argument that SES domains differ across age and gender groups and supporting arguments for the use of age- and gender-specific indexes in studies of health inequalities. Such a focus on specific population groups is particularly relevant for women. Women's increasing labor force participation, accompanied by growing numbers of female-headed families and the decline of fertility rates, challenges the traditional assumptions that the male breadwinner is the determinant of a household's socio-economic position

(Hayes & Jones, 1992). In the late 1980s, fewer women in their 50s than in their 40s were in paid work, and they tended to work from financial necessity (Arber & Ginn, 1995). Research suggests that this may be changing and that many women now in this age group are more ambitious than men of similar age (Bradley, 1998). Many young Australian women perceive a combination of motherhood and paid work to be the norm and aspire to such a lifestyle by the age of 35 (Wicks & Mishra, 1997). Despite their increasing participation in the paid workforce, women today still perform the majority of domestic and caring work (Bittman, 1995). Women are likely to be engaged in multiple social roles related to paid employment, family, child-care, and caring for others (Pugh & Moser, 1990); their lives thus remain markedly different from those of men. The need for gender-specific measures of SES, particularly those that take sociocultural factors into account, is therefore critical. In addition, factors such as delayed retirement and self-funded retirement will increasingly impinge on the material well being of older women. The "complex mosaic" (Mowl & Turner, 1995) of women's lives as they move through different life stages calls for more sensitive measures of SES to take account of this diversity.

Gender differences in health vary according to stage of the life cycle (Arber & Cooper, 1999) and increasing evidence suggests that socio-economic factors acting over the lifetime may have cumulative effects on health (Hart et al., 1998; Smith, Hart, Blane, Gillis & Hawthorne, 1997). The longitudinal nature of the WHA study affords the opportunity to further explore, over time, the marked difference between the age groups in regard to the influence of paid employment. Will continued participation in paid work through their young and middle years affect the SES of women after retirement? Will employment remain less relevant to older women? Or is the association demonstrated in this study a generational effect specific to these cohorts, derived from the fact that the mid-aged women have typically engaged in some form of paid work while the other older group has not?

Associations between the type of family unit and women's health require further investigation. Evidence from British studies suggests that differences between never-married women and divorced and separated women may vary by age and/or birth cohort. Among older British women, divorced and separated women may have experienced more harmful health effects than never-married women; however, among younger women, this difference may be absent or possibly reversed (Waldron, Weiss, & Hughes, 1997). The longitudinal WHA study affords opportunities to examine these associations over time for Australian women.

Strengths of this study include the large, representative population samples of women surveyed and the comprehensive range of health indicators assessed. Limitations include the fact that only those socio-economic and demographic items included in the WHA surveys could be included in analyses. Other potentially important proxies for SES, such as inherited wealth or material possessions, may have altered the factor structure if they had been included. In addition, early life SES, which emerging evidence suggests plays a key role in contributing to health inequalities throughout life (e.g., Power & Matthews, 1997; Wamala, Lynch, & Kaplan, 2001), was not assessed comprehensively in this study. The data presented are cross-sectional, and hence results of the investigation described in this article demonstrate associations only. However, again the longitudinal WHA study provides great potential for future exploration of causal connections and the cumulative effects of SES on health over time, and in the context of significant life events. For example, what is the effect of children leaving home? Does the removal of such a demand on parental resources mean that housing unit becomes less relevant as a contribution to SES?

These findings add to the growing body of evidence demonstrating links between low SES and poor health and indicate that these associations differ depending on the domain of SES and the age group under study. The finding that different SES domains were differently associated with health outcomes across age groups suggests that underlying relations between SES and health are likely to be complex and governed by different mechanisms depending partly on age and aspect of health. Further research is required to untangle these complex patterns and investigate the causal mechanisms between SES and health outcomes. A better understanding of these causal pathways is critical to begin to address SES-related health inequalities.

REFERENCES

Anderson, R. T., Sorlie, P., Backlund, E., Johnson, N., & Kaplan, G. A. (1997). Mortality effects of community socioeconomic status. *Epidemiology, 8,* 42–47.

Arber, S. (1997). Comparing inequalities in women's and men's health: Britain in the 1990s. *Social Science and Medicine, 44,* 773–787.

Arber, S., & Ginn, J. (1995). The mirage of gender equality: Occupational success in the labour market and within marriage. *British Journal of Sociology, 46,* 21–43.

Arber S., & Cooper, H. (1999). Gender differences in health in later life: The new paradox? *Social Science and Medicine, 48,* 61–76.S

Australian Bureau of Statistics. (1995). *National Health Survey: User's guide* (Catalogue No. 4363.0). Canberra: Australian Bureau of Statistics.

Australian Bureau of Statistics. (1999). *Labour force status and other characteristics of migrants, Australia* (Catalogue No. 6250.0). Canberra: Australian Government Publishing Service.

Austrialian National Health and Medical Research Council. (1997). *Acting on Australia's weight: A strategic plan for the prevention of overweight and obesity.* Canberra: Australian Government Publishing Service.

Baghurst, K. I., Record, S. J., Baghurst, P. A., Syrette, J. A., Crawford, D., & Worsley, A. (1990). Sociodemographic determinants in Australia of the intake of food and nutrients implicated in cancer aetiology. *The Medical Journal of Australia, 153,* 444–452.

Baxter, J. (1991). The class location of women: Direct or derived? In J. Baxter & M. Western (Eds.), *Class analysis and contemporary Australia* (pp. 202–222). South Melbourne: MacMillan.

Berkman, C. S., & Gurland, B. J. (1998). The relationship among income, other socioeconomic indicators, and functional level in older persons. *Journal of Aging and Health, 10,* 81–98.

Bittman, M. (1995). Recent changes in unpaid work (Occasional Paper, ABS Catalogue No. 4154.0). Canberra: Australian Bureau of Statistics.

Bradley, H. (1998). A new gendered order? Researching and rethinking women's work. *Sociology, 33,* 869–873.

Brezinka, V., & Kittel, F. (1996). Psychosocial factors of coronary heart disease in women: A review. *Social Science & Medicine, 42,* 1351–1365.

Broom, D. H. (1984). The social distribution of illness: Is Australia more equal? *Social Science and Medicine, 18,* 909–917.

Brown, W. J., Bryson, L. B., Byles, J. E., Dobson, A. J., Lee, C., Mishra, G., & Schofield, M. (1998). Women's Health Australia: Recruitment for a national longitudinal cohort study. *Women and Health, 28,* 23–40.

Brown, W. J., Mishra, G., Lee, C., & Bauman, A. (2000). Leisure time physical activity in Australian women: Relationship with well-being and symptoms. *Research Quarterly for Exercise and Sport, 71,* 206–216.

Chandola, T. (2000). Social class differences in mortality using the new UK national statistics socio-economic classification. *Social Science and Medicine, 50,* 641–649.

Crespo, C. J., Ainsworth, B. E., Keteyian, S. J., Heath, G. W., & Smit, E. (1999). Prevalence of physical inactivity and its relation to social class in U.S. adults: Results from the Third National Health and Nutrition Examination Survey, 1988–1994. *Medicine and Science in Sports and Exercise, 31,* 1821–1827.

Daniel, A. (1984). The measurement of social class. *Community Health Studies, 8,* 218–222.

Der, G., MacIntyre, S., Ford, G., Hunt, K., & West, P. (1999). The relationship of household income to a range of health measures in three age cohorts from the West of Scotland. *European Journal of Public Health, 9,* 271–277.

Elo, I. T., & Preston, S. H. (1996). Educational differentials in mortality: United States, 1979–1985. *Social Science & Medicine, 42,* 47–57.

Evans, J. M. M., Newton, R. W., Ruta, D. A., MacDonald, T. M., & Morris, A. D. (2000). Socio-economic status, obesity, and prevalence of Type 1 and Type 2 diabetes mellitus. *Diabetic Medicine, 17,* 478–480.

Graham, H., & Hunt, S. (1994). Women's smoking and measures of women's socioeconomic status in the United Kingdom. *Health Promotion International, 9,* 81–88.

Hair, J. F., Jr., Anderson, R. E., Tatham R. L., & Black, W. C. (1997). *Multivariate data analysis with readings* (4th ed.). Upper Saddle River, NJ: Prentice Hall International Editions.

Hallqvist, J., Lundbert, M., Diderichsen, F., & Ahlbom, A. (1998). Socioeconomic differences in risk of myocardial infarction 1971–1994 in Sweden: Time trends, relative risks, and population attributable risks. *International Journal of Epidemiology, 27,* 410–415.

Hart, C. L., Davey Smith G., & Blane D. (1998). Inequalities in mortality by social class measured at three stages of the life course. *American Journal of Public Health, 88,* 471–474.

Hayes, B., & Jones, F. (1992). Class identification among Australian couples: Are wives' characteristics relevant? *British Journal of Sociology, 43,* 463–484.

Hemingway, H., Nicholson, A., Stafford, M., Roberts, R., & Marmot, M. (1997). The impact of socioeconomic status on health functioning as assessed by the SF-36 questionnaire: The Whitehall 2 study. *American Journal of Public Health, 87,* 1484–1490.

House, J., Lepkowski, J., Kinney, A., Mero, R. Kessler, R., & Herzog, A. (1994). The social stratification of aging and health. *Journal of Health and Social Behaviour, 35,* 213–34.

Johanson, J. F., & Sonnenberg, A. (1990). The prevalence of hemorrhoids and chronic constipation: An epidemiologic study. *Gastroenterology, 98,* 380–386.

Kline, P. (1994). An easy guide to factor analysis. London: Routledge.

Koskinen, S., & Martelin, T. (1994). Why are socioeconomic mortality differences smaller among women than among men? *Social Science and Medicine, 38,* 1385–1396.

Kreiger, N. (2000). Refiguring "race": Epidemiology, racialized biology, and biological expressions of race relations. International Journal of Health Services, 30, 211–216.

Kreiger, N., Williams, D., & Moss, N. (1997). Measuring social class in U.S. public health research: Concepts, methodologies, and guidelines. *Annual Review of Public Health, 18,* 341–378.

Liberatos, P., Link, B. G., & Kelsey, J. L. (1988). The measurement of social class in epidemiology. *Epidemiology Review, 10,* 87–122.

Mackenbach, J. P. (1992). Socio-economic health differences in the Netherlands: A review of recent empirical findings. *Social Science & Medicine, 34,* 213–226.

Martikainen, P. (1995). Mortality and socio-economic status among Finnish women. *Population Studies, 49,* 71–90.

McDonough, P., Williams, D. R., House, J. S., & Duncan, G. J. (1999). Gender and the socioeconomic gradient in mortality. *Journal of Health and Social Behaviour, 40,* 17–31.

McElduff, P., & Dobson, A. J. (2000). Trends in coronary heart disease: Has the socio-economic differential changed? *Australian and New Zealand Journal of Public Health, 24,* 465–473.

Mishra, G. D., Ball, K., Dobson, A. J., Byles, J. E., & Warner-Smith, P. (2001). The measurement of socioeconomic status: Investigation of gender- and age-specific indicators in Australia: National Health Survey '95. *Social Indicators Research, 56,* 73–89.

Mowl, G., & Towner, J. (1995). Women, gender, leisure, and place: Towards a more humanistic geography of women's leisure. *Leisure Studies, 14,* 102–116.

Mustard, C. A., Derksen, S., Bethelot, J. M., Wolfson, M., & Roos, L. L. (1997). Age-specific education and income gradients in morbidity and mortality in a Canadian province. *Social Science and Medicine, 45,* 383–397.

Neter, J., Kutner, M. H., Nachtsheim, C. J., & Wasserman, W. (1996). *Applied linear statistical model.* Chicago: Irwin.

Osler, M., Gerdes, L. U., Davidsen, M., Bronnum-Hansen, H., Madsen, M., Jorgensen, T., & Schroll, M. (2000). Socioeconomic status and trends in risk factors for cardiovascular diseases in the Danish MONICA population, 1982–1992. *Journal of Epidemiology & Community Health, 54,* 108–113.

Power, C., & Matthews, S. (1997). Origins of health inequalities in a national population sample. *Lancet, 350,* 1584–1589.

Pugh, H., & Moser, K. (1990). Measuring women's mortality differences. In H. Roberts (Ed.), *Women's health counts* (pp. 93–112). London: Routledge.

Robert, S., & House, J. (1996). SES differentials in health by age and alternative indicators of SES. *Journal of Aging and Health, 8,* 359–388.

Sarlio-Lahteenkorva, S., & Lahelma, E. (1999). The association of body mass index with social and economic disadvantage in women and men. *International Journal of Epidemiology, 28,* 445–449.

SAS Institute Inc. (1989). SAS/STAT user's guide (Version 6, 4th ed., Vol. 2). Cary, NC: Author.

Scambler, G., & Higgs, P. (1999). Stratification, class, and health: Class relations and health inequalities in high modernity. *Sociology, 33,* 275–288.

Smith, G. D., Hart, C., Blane, D., Gillis, C., & Hawthorne, V. (1997). Lifetime socioeconomic position and mortality: Prospective observational study. *British Medical Journal, 314,* 547–552.

Sobal, J., & Stunkard, A. J. (1989). Socioeconomic status and obesity: A review of the literature. *Psychological Bulletin, 105,* 260–275.

Tyroler, H. A. (1999). The influence of socioeconomic factors on cardiovascular disease risk factor development. *Preventive Medicine, 29*(Suppl. S), S36–S40.

Vargas, C. M., Ingram, D. D., & Gillum, R. F. (2000). Incidence of hypertension and educational attainment: The NHANES I epidemiologic follow-up study. First National Health and Nutrition Examination Survey. *American Journal of Epidemiology, 152,* 272–278.

Waldron, I., Weiss, C. C., & Hughes, M. E. (1997). Marital status effects on health: Are there differences between never married women and divorced and separated women? *Social Science & Medicine, 45,* 1387–1397.

Wamala, S. P., Lynch, J., & Kaplan, G. A. (2001). Women's exposure to early and later life socioeconomic disadvantage and coronary heart disease risk: The Stockholm Female Coronary Risk Study. *International Journal of Epidemiology, 30,* 275–284.

Ware, J. E., Kosinski, M., & Keller, S. D. (1994). SF–36 physical and mental health summary scales: A user's manual. Boston: The Health Institute, New England Medical Center.

Weber, M. (1946). Class, status, and party. In H. Gerth & W. W. Mills (Eds.), *From Max Weber: Essays in sociology (pp. 180–195).* New York: Oxford University Press.

Wicks, D., & Mishra, G. (1997). Young Australian women and their aspirations for work, education, and relationships. In E. Carson, A. Jamrozik, & T. Winefield (Eds.), *Unemployment: Economic promise and political will* (pp. 89–100). London: Academic.

Young, A. F., Dobson, A. J., & Byles, J. E. (2001). Determinants of general practitioner use among women in Australia. *Social Science and Medicine, 53,* 1641–1651.

INTERNATIONAL JOURNAL OF BEHAVIORAL MEDICINE, 9(3), 286–300

Causal Explanations for Common Somatic Symptoms Among Women and Men

Karin Nykvist, Anders Kjellberg, and Carina Bildt

The purpose of this study was to examine categories of causal attributions assessed by women and men regarding common somatic symptoms. A questionnaire was sent out to a randomly selected sample of 1,500 persons followed by a screening of respondents with symptom experience. To identify groups of individuals considering different causes or causal categories as important, separate cluster analyses were made of ratings for neck/shoulder problems and sore/upset stomach. The results showed similarities between assessed causal categories for the two types of symptoms and that women in this sample were overrepresented, particularly in considering psychological explanations for their symptoms, whereas the men were overrepresented in not considering any of the causes as particularly important. This was discussed in terms of illness severity and an association between psychological and somatic distress in people's experience, such as stress and total workload, and in their subsequent explanatory models suggesting differences in beliefs about a connection between body and mind.

Key words: causal explanations, somatic symptoms, women and men

There are a variety of ways to perceive and think about illness, state of health, and symptoms in people's everyday thinking. This may be reflected in individuals' different beliefs, assumptions, interpretations, and causal explanations of their illnesses or symptoms. Everyday thinking is influenced by, for example, past experience and medical history, type of experienced illness or symptom, individual

Karin Nykvist, Anders Kjellberg, and Carina Bildt, National Institute for Working Life, Stockholm, Sweden.

Correspondence for this article should be sent to Karin Nykvist, National Institute for Working Life, S–11279, Stockholm, Sweden. E-mail: Karin.Nykvist@niwl.se disposition, and the knowledge and beliefs that exist in a society at a specific time. The most notable features in everyday thinking of disease found by Blaxter (1983) among working-class women in Scotland were the salience given to knowing the cause, the striving for rational explanation, and the importance of linking together life events. In a study of concepts of health, Blaxter (1990) found that women at all ages, in general, gave more expansive answers than men. Women showed a stronger tendency to express many-dimensional concepts of health and were rather more likely than men to locate psychological factors, family structures, and social relationships as being important influences on health. In a study by Walters (1993), stress was shown to be a central theme among women when asked to identify their three main health problems.

There may be differences in causal explanations for diseases and physical symptoms. Disease often has a label or diagnosis attached. Symptoms are not necessarily associated with a distinct disease and are more commonly open to a variety of interpretations. Physical symptoms, for example, can be attributed to minor transient causes, stress, or psychological factors or to a potentially serious disease. The decision about what to do with a symptom (e.g., ignore it; consult a doctor) may partly depend on what the individual believes is the cause of the symptom (Robbins & Kirmayer, 1991).

Robbins and Kirmayer (1991) identified three dimensions of causal attributions for physical symptoms: physical illness ("somatic"), emotional distress ("psychological") and environmental events ("external"). They found that women scored significantly higher on the psychological attribution scale than men, but not on the somatic or external scale. Women reported more somatic complaints that had no immediate organic diagnosis.

Individuals who strongly endorse one set of causes tend to endorse other causal explanations as well. Robbins and Kirmayer (1991) found moderate intercorrelations among the attribution scales. They suggest that this may reflect an association between psychological and somatic distress both in people's experience and in their subsequent explanatory models. Individuals who include psychological factors in their explanations of somatic symptoms may subscribe to more complex causal models, which also include somatic, psychosocial, and external factors.

In summary, the main purpose of this study was to examine gender differences in causal attributions for common somatic symptoms. Considering the female excess of symptom reporting (e.g., Gijsbers van Wijk, Van-Vliet, Kolk, & Everaerd, 1991; Verbrugge, 1985, 1989), a secondary question of interest was whether causal attributions were influenced by the duration for which the symptom was experienced.

METHOD

A questionnaire was sent out to a random sample of 1,500 Swedes (750 men and 750 women) between the ages of 25 and 55. The random selected names were obtained from the Swedish company Sema-Group Infodata AB. One reminder letter, followed by a new copy of the questionnaire, was sent after 3 weeks to those who had failed to return the questionnaire.

Response Rate and Generalizability

Complete data were obtained from 678 persons (399 women and 279 men). The nonresponse rate was particularly high among men (response: men = 37%; women = 53%). There were no notable differences in the response rate between age groups. In the three age groups (25–35, 36–45, and 46–55), the response rate was 46,% 42%, and 47%, respectively. Neither were there any differences in the age distribution between men and women answering the questionnaire (χ^2 = 2.58, df = 2, p = .275).

Table 1 presents a comparison on selected characteristics between participants in the sample and in the general Swedish population. The respondents had a significantly higher educational level than that observed in the general population, but there were no differences between the men and women within the sample (χ^2 = 2.31, df = 2, p = .315). The male respondents had the same level of workforce participation as that of the general population, but the female respondents had a slightly higher workforce participation than the general population. Within the sample, there was a

TABLE 1
Level of Education, Workforce Participation, and Civil Status (%)
in the Swedish Population and in the Sample

	*Population (%)		Sample (%)		χ^2 Value (Population vs. Sample)	
	Men	Women	Men	Women	Men	Women
Level of education[a]					7.8**	19.1*
Compulsory school	19	15	17	16		
Upper secondary	52	53	46	41		
Higher education	29	32	37	43		
Workforce participation[b]					1,2***	7.8**
Full-time	82	57	81	50		
Part-time	4	24	5	28		
Not in workforce	14	19	14	22		
Civil status[c]					13.7*	40.1*
Married/cohabiting	58	62	68	78		
Single	42	38	32	22		

[a]Source = Swedish statistics, 1999. [b]Source = Swedish statistics, 2000, 1998. [c]Source = Swedish statistics, 1998.
*p <.001. **p < .005. ***ns.

significant difference in workforce participation between men and women ($\chi^2 = 73.02$, $df = 2$, $p < .001$). The respondents were more frequently married or cohabiting than those in the general population. Within the sample, women were significantly more frequently married or cohabiting than the men ($\chi^2 = 7.58$, $df = 1$, $p = .006$).

To get an indication of the representativity of the sample with regard to health status, the proportion of men and women reporting their health as less good ("*neither good or bad*," "*bad*," or "*very bad*") was compared to corresponding data from a health survey in the county of Stockholm in 1998 (see Table 2; Folkhälsorapport, 1999).

There was a somewhat higher proportion of persons reporting their health as less good among the respondents in this study than among the respondents in the Stockholm health survey, particularly among the male respondents.

All respondents were categorized according to type of symptom experienced. Neck/shoulder problems were experienced by 66% of the respondents (170 men and 275 women). Slightly more respondents from the 25 to 35 age group (166 respondents) than from the older age groups (124 and 155 respondents, respectively) experienced these symptoms. Sore/upset stomach was reported by 49% of the respondents (139 men and 192 women). Slightly more respondents from the 25 to 35 age group (137 respondents) than from the two older age groups (90 and 104 respondents, respectively) experienced these symptoms.

Measures

Respondents were asked to rate the likelihood of 29 different causes for their symptoms. Each cause was rated on a 7-point Likert-type scale ranging from 0 (*completely without importance*) to 6 (*very important cause*).

Twenty one of these causes were exactly the same for the two types of problems (Table 3) and consisted of 6 items referring to somatic causes, 8 items referring to psychological (personal) causes, 3 items referring to work situation, and 4 items referring to private situation apart from work. These items were also subdivided into causes regarded as stable or more temporary in character, such as being a worrying

TABLE 2
Percentage of Men and Women Reporting Less Than Good Health According
to Age in a Health Survey in Stockholm and in This Sample

Health Survey in Stockholm (%)[a]				*Sample (%) (All Respondents)*			
Men		*Women*		*Men*		*Women*	
20–44	45–64	20–44	45–64	25–44	45–55	25–44	45–55
12	21	14	20	16	27	16	23

[a]Source = Public health report for Stockholm 1999.

TABLE 3
Mean Ratings Per Cluster of Causal Items Regarding Neck and Shoulder Symptoms and t Tests of the Sex Difference for Each Item

Causal Item	Eight-Cluster Solution of Neck and Shoulder								Total[a]	Women[b]	Men[c]	t	p
	1	2	3	4	5	6	7	8					
Work situation													
Physically strained work situation	2.43	3.35	2.38	.85	.61	3.57	4.13	4.52	2.03	2.12	1.87	1.13	.258
Psychologically strained work situation	1.17	3.35	3.88	1.98	.80	4.16	1.46	3.06	1.91	2.06	1.67	1.95	.052
Temporary problems at work	.60	2.88	2.88	1.28	.24	2.67	.94	1.00	1.10	1.23	.88	2.20	.029
Private situation													
Physically strained private situation	.75	3.82	1.74	.90	.33	1.69	.69	.82	.90	.92	.87	0.31	.753
Psychologically strained private situation	.45	4.18	4.50	1.69	.40	1.84	.25	.21	1.12	1.29	.84	2.89	.004
Temporary private problems	.17	3.00	3.54	1.34	.18	1.41	.38	.33	.83	.89	.73	1.15	.250
Strained life situation	.25	3.21	3.19	1.31	.12	1.17	.27	.06	.74	.77	.69	0.61	.542

(Continued)

TABLE 3
(CONTINUED)

Psychological causes													
Worried as a person	.15	3.30	2.91	1.40	.17	2.07	.02	.33	.85	.89	.77	0.87	.385
Temporarily worried	.24	3.76	4.81	2.22	.43	2.91	.54	.39	1.36	1.56	1.03	3.14	.002
Having high demands on oneself	1.15	4.18	5.00	3.09	.73	4.04	.13	3.64	2.04	2.31	1.59	3.52	.000
Taking on too much responsibility	1.37	4.35	4.50	3.21	.76	4.08	.50	3.61	2.10	2.42	1.58	4.23	.000
Have as a person difficulties relaxing	1.00	4.56	4.65	2.69	.66	3.65	.29	1.27	1.73	1.91	1.43	2.54	.011
Have temporary difficulties to relax	.33	3.99	4.58	2.55	.64	3.25	.46	.70	1.54	1.80	1.13	3.68	.000
General psychological sensitivity	.30	3.35	3.77	1.48	.21	1.61	.15	.24	.89	1.00	.71	2.04	.042
Temporarily psychological unfit	.10	3.03	4.14	1.55	.20	1.98	.29	.58	.98	1.10	.77	2.26	.024

(Continued)

TABLE 3
(Continued)

Eight-Cluster Solution of Neck and Shoulder

	1	2	3	4	5	6	7	8	Total[a]	Women[b]	Men[c]	t	p
Physical causes													
General physical sensitivity	1.31	*4.53*	1.85	1.39	2.08	1.00	.94	1.33	84	.89	1.60	-4.67	.000
Temporarily physically unfit	.25	*3.24*	*2.88*	1.01	.47	1.57	,48	.73	,92	1.07	.69	2.78	.006
Temporary sensitive muscles/stomach	.73	*4.35*	*3.00*	1.22	.93	*2.84*	1,90	.94	1.53	1.62	1.39	1.30	.196
Longstanding sickness	*5.30*	*4.53*	.38	.45	.05	.82	.27	.17	.89	1.01	.71	1.65	.101
Temporary sickness/injury	.71	*4.06*	1.08	.29	.38	1.50	1.75	.71	.88	.93	.79	0.91	.362
Age	.82	3.71	1.85	.88	.36	1.88	1.04	1.45	1.02	1.04	1.00	0.26	.792

Note. Italicized = mean values 2.0 total mean. Cluster labeling: Cluster 1 (40 cases) = Longstanding sickness; Cluster 2 (17 cases) = Almost all causes; Cluster 3 (26 cases),4 (67 cases);and 6 (51 cases)= Psychological causes; Cluster 5 (163 cases) = No particular cause important; and Cluster 7 (48 cases);8 (33 cases) = Physical work situation (symptom specific).
[a]N = 445. [b]n = 275. [c]n = 170.

TABLE 4
Percentage Belonging to the Eight Neck/Shoulder and Stomach Clusters and the Percentage Reporting Long Symptom Duration

	Percentage of Cases per Cluster			Symptom Duration per Cluster (%)	
Neck/Shoulder and Stomach Clusters	Total	Women	Men	Occasionally	LongTime < 2 Weeks
Neck/shoulder[a]					
1. Longstanding sickness	9	10	7	10	90
Psychological causes					
4. Demands/responsibility (slightly important)	15	16	13	70	30
6. Psychological work situation and demands	12	14	7	34	66
3. Private situation and psychological causes	6	7	4	50	50
2. Somatic and Psychological causes (almost all causes)	4	4	4	19	81
5. Nothing particularly important	37	31	46	68	32
Symptom specific					
7. Physical work situation	11	9	14	60	40
8. Physical work situation and demands/responsibility	7	9	5	36	64
Total percentage	100	100	100	53	47
Stomach[b]					
1. Longstanding sickness	4	4	4	8	92
Psychological causes					
4. Demands/responsibility (slightly important)	22	24	19	65	35
6. Psychological work situation and psychological causes	3	5	1	50	50
3. Private situation, demands/responsibility and relaxing	9	11	5	24	76
2. Somatic and Psychological causes (almost all causes)	5	6	4	37	63
5. Nothing particularly important	40	29	54	80	20
Symptom specific					
7. Worried/difficulties to relax as a person	14	16	11	31	69
8. Temporarily worried and psychological unfit	5	2	58	42	4
Total percentage	100	100	100	58	42

[a]$N = 445$. [b]$N = 331$.

person or temporarily worried, respectively. The remaining items with differences in the formulation for the two types of problems, thus not comparable, referred to behavioral causes, such as too little exercise and unhealthy habits, and external causes, such as weather/draft and dirty kitchens/shops.

In addition to the 29 items, the questionnaire included an open-ended question about other important causes and a question about the duration (occasional, several weeks, months, or years) of symptom experience for neck/shoulder and stomach problems, respectively.

The respondents were also asked about their beliefs regarding the connection between their mental well-being and physical state. The respondents were asked two questions: "Does your mental well-being affect your physical state?" and " Does your physical state effect your mental well-being?" that they rated on a scale ranging from 0 (*no, not at all*) to 6 (*yes, very much*). An index was calculated as means of the ratings of two questions about associations between mental and physical state.

The questionnaire also included measures of symptom reporting, body awareness, body dissatisfaction, negative affect, self-esteem, illness behavior, and self-rated health, which will be presented elsewhere.

Statistical Analyses

To identify groups of individuals considering different causes or causal categories as important, separate cluster analyses were made of the neck/shoulder and stomach ratings. Ward's method, with squared Euclidean distances, was used for these analyses, which included the 21 causal items common for neck/shoulder symptoms (Table 3) and symptoms from the stomach.

RESULTS

Causal Items of Importance

The results showed that women rated a higher number of causes as important (a rating of 4 or more) compared to men. Mean number of causes rated as important for neck/shoulder problems was 4.92 for women and 3.81 for men ($t = 2.38, df = 431, p = .018$) and 5.29 and 3.77, respectively, for causes of stomach problems ($t = 2.70, df = 17, p = .008$). Women and men were relatively in agreement regarding the causes considered most important. Both women and men regarded high demands, taking on too much responsibility, and a strained work situation to be the most important causes for neck and shoulder problems (Table 3). Taking on too much responsibility and having high demands on oneself were, however, also causes that women rated significantly more important than men regarding neck/shoulder (Table 3). This gender difference was also shown regarding stomach problems ($t = 4.5, t = 4.3$, respectively, $p < .001$). Mean ratings for taking on too much responsibility and having high demands on oneself were 2.70 and 2.81, respectively, for women and 1.68 and 1.82, respectively, for men. The opposite gender difference was found for the rated importance of general physical sensitivity for neck and shoulder problems, but not for stomach problems.

Women and men were also relatively in agreement about the importance regarding the behavioral and external causes that were not completely comparable between neck/shoulder problems and stomach problems. Too little exercise and bad working technique were regarded as the most important causes of neck/shoulder problems by both women ($M = 2.84$ and $M = 2.43$, respectively) and men ($M = 2.22$ and $M = 1.85$, respectively). These two causes were also the ones that showed significant gender differences ($t = 3.00, t = 2.90$, respectively, $p = .003$). Temporary negligence of sleep or food was considered as the most important of the behavioral and external causes of stomach problems among both women ($M = 2.06$) and men ($M = 2.11$). The small gender difference was not significant ($t = -0.20, p = .708$).

The mean rating of the influence of the psychological well-being on the physical well-being was higher for women ($M = 4.39, SD = 1.27$) than for men ($M = 3.98, SD = 1.2, t = 3.24, df = 430, p = .001$). This rating was moderately correlated with the number of causes judged to be important ($r = .287, p < .001$).

Cluster Analysis of Causal Attributions of Neck and Shoulder Problems

An eight-cluster solution was chosen for the causal items regarding neck/shoulder problems. As shown in Table 3, the cluster analysis yielded one cluster referring to longstanding illness (Cluster 1), three clusters referring to psychological causes (Cluster 3, 4, and 6), one cluster assessing almost all causes as important (Cluster 2), and another not considering any particular cause important (Cluster 5). Clusters 7 and 8 were both characterized by physically strained work situation. The members of Cluster 8 also had rather high ratings of the items high demands/responsibility and psychologically strained work situation.

The distribution of women and men differed significantly between the clusters ($\chi^2 = 19.0, df = 7, p = .008$). In Cluster 5 (none of the causes important) and Cluster 7 (physical work situation), men were overrepresented (Table 4), whereas they were underrepresented in five of the clusters: Cluster 1 (illness), Cluster 3 (private situation and psychological causes), Cluster 4 (high demands/responsibility), Cluster 6 (psychological work situation and high demands), and Cluster 8 (physical work situation and high demands/responsibility).

Members of the clusters referring to psychological causes had significantly ($t = 2.98, df = 176, p = .003$) stronger beliefs ($M = 4.54, SD = 1.15$) about an association between psychological and physical well-being than members of the cluster referring to longstanding illness ($M = 3.86, SD = 1.51$). Furthermore, respondents referring to almost all causes showed slightly stronger beliefs ($M = 4.59, SD = 1.01$) about such an association than did respondents who did not consider any particular cause ($M = 4.03, SD = 1.23$), although the difference was not significant ($t = 1.94, df = 73, p = .067$).

Cluster Analysis of Causal Attributions of Stomach Problems

The cluster analysis of the causal items regarding stomach problems yielded an eight-cluster solution where the first five clusters were virtually identical with the neck/shoulder clusters. Cluster 6 was characterized by high ratings of all items referring to psychological causes, whereas Clusters 7 and 8 had high ratings of stable and temporary psychological characteristics, respectively.

As for neck/shoulder problems, men were overrepresented in Cluster 5 (none of the causes important) and underrepresented in the five psychological clusters as well as in the cluster where almost all causes was considered important (Table 4).

Although the cluster solutions for neck/shoulder and stomach problems were very similar, the association between cluster memberships in the two cluster analyses was rather weak ($\kappa = .275$).

In the group that answered both the neck and stomach questions, 46% of the women and 26% of the men belonged to one of the three psychological neck/shoulder clusters (3, 4, and 6). Corresponding figures for the psychological stomach clusters (3, 4, 6, 7, and 8) were 61% and 34%.

Attributions and Duration of Symptom Experience

The distribution of women and men differed significantly in reported length of symptom experience for neck/shoulder problems ($\chi^2 = 15.6, df = 1, p < .001$) and for stomach problems ($\chi^2 = 4.7, df = 1, p = .030$). Fifty four percent of the women reported a long (several weeks, months, years) duration of their neck/shoulder problems in contrast to 35% of the men. Forty seven percent of the women reported a long duration of their stomach problems in contrast to 35% of the men.

As shown in Table 4, in the clusters in which men were overrepresented (none of the causes important and physical work), a large proportion of respondents reported only occasional day or days experience of their problems. In contrast, a large proportion of respondents considering almost all causes important reported a long duration of their problems. In the psychological clusters overrepresented by women, a long duration of their symptoms was foremost reported by members in Cluster 6 (psychological work situation and high demands) regarding neck/shoulder and members in Cluster 3 (private situation and psychological causes) and Cluster 7 (worried as a person) regarding stomach problems. As would be expected, the majority of respondents referring to long-standing sickness also reported a long duration of their problems.

Other Causes of Importance

In addition to the causal items, the questionnaire included an open-ended question about other important causes. Forty seven women and 28 men reported other important causes apart from or in addition to the rated explanatory items regarding neck/shoulder problems and 31 women compared to 12 men regarding stomach problems. Most of the additional causes mentioned were a specification of the rated explanatory items. For example, respondents who mentioned work-related additional causes, such as computer- and monotonous work, also had high ratings on the explanatory item work technique and all of the cases mentioning stress (8% of the women) had high ratings of the psychological explanatory items. Additional causes mentioned that were not corresponding to the rated explanatory items were relatively gender-related causes referring to sports/leisure (14% of the men and 4% of the women) and pregnancy/child-care (3% of the men and 13% of the women).

CONCLUSIONS AND DISCUSSION

In this study we set out to examine causal explanations of common somatic symptoms and whether women and men attributed their symptoms to different causal categories.

A comparison between the eight-cluster solutions for neck/shoulder and stomach problems showed similarities between assessed causal categories for the two types of somatic problems. The main difference was seen in the two last clusters. For stomach symptoms these two clusters were characterized by psychological causes, whereas the clusters regarding neck/shoulder referred to physical work situation.

A larger part of the women belonged to clusters referring to psychological causes. Men were overrepresented in the cluster not considering any of the causes important and in the cluster that rated physical work as the solely important cause for neck and shoulder problems.

One possible interpretation of the relatively large group that did not consider any of the causal categories as particularly important is that some causes that are particularly important for men were not included in the questionnaire. However, the answers to the open-ended question about causes give no indication that this would be the case. Most of the causes added by the respondents could be regarded as specifications of the more general causal categories given in the questionnaire. Furthermore, more men than women could be expected to answer the open-ended question, if there was a neglected causal category more important for men, but the proportion of men was similar to the proportion of women that reported additional important causes. A more likely interpretation, when considering that a very large amount of these respondents reported only occasional experience of the two types of symptoms, is that the respondents who did not judge any of the causes as important represented a relatively healthy group of people who therefore did not find it necessary to refer their symptoms to any specific cause. In contrast, a large amount of the respondents who considered almost all causes as important reported a long duration of their symptom and a possible interpretation is, thus, that these respondents represent a group with more serious but undiagnosed somatic problems.

The low response rate makes the representativity of the sample questionable. The biased sampling was confirmed by a comparison between the sample and the general population. The relative sizes of different subgroups (e.g., groups showing different attributional patterns) are thus probably biased. The larger proportion of both women and men that was married or lived together may, for example, have had such an effect on the results. However, a more important question in this context is whether such a bias is likely to have caused an over or underestimation of the sex differences. One indication that this might have been the case is that there was a slightly higher proportion of women working part-time and not participating in the workforce in the sample, compared to the general population. This may, for example, have influenced the judged importance of causal categories, total workload, and levels of stress. Furthermore, persons reporting their health as less good seem to have been somewhat overrepresented in the sample, particularly among the male respondents, which might indicate an underestimation rather than an overestimation of differences between men and women in this study regarding reported duration of their symptoms.

There is probably no single explanation as to why somatic symptoms are attributed to psychological causes. Possibly, experiences of high levels of stress make a person more likely to acknowledge that somatic symptoms can be an expression of psychological distress. If so, such experiences should be more common among women. A study by Lundberg, Mårdberg, and Frankenhauser (1994) indicated that this might be true because they found that women, by having the main responsibility for family and home, had a higher total workload in terms of hours per week. A work overload accompanied by high levels of stress may also induce symptoms such as musculoskeletal disorders (Lundberg, 1996) and probably also symptoms from the stomach. The differences between men's and women's life situation shown by these and other studies may explain the overrepresentation of women among respondents considering a strained work situation and having high demands on oneself as important causes of their neck/shoulder problem. The overrepresentation of women who considered a psychologically strained private situation, high demands, and difficulty relaxing as important causes of their stomach problem may have the same background.

An interesting aspect shown by Blaxter's (1990) study was that women showed a stronger tendency to express many-dimensional concepts of health and were rather more likely than men to locate psychological factors, family structures, and social relationships as being important influences on health. Another interesting feature of women's thinking of their diseases pointed out by Blaxter (1983) was the importance of linking together life events. Thus, a many-dimensional or multifactorial explanatory model may also indicate that the different types of causes are regarded as causally linked together. There were, for example, a larger proportion of women than men linking together a physically strained work situation, having high demands, and taking on too much responsibility regarding their neck/shoulder problem, whereas a larger proportion of the men considered solely physical work situation important.

Our results also showed that women rated a larger number of causes as important compared to men. Furthermore, the rated number of important causes was related to the deemed importance of psychological factors for somatic symptoms. These results indicate an association between psychological and multifactorial explanatory models for somatic symptoms and that such models are more common among women than men.

In summary, the results show that women in this sample were overrepresented in considering psychological explanations for their somatic symptoms, whereas men were overrepresented in not considering any of the causes as particularly important. This was discussed in terms of seriousness of illness and the association between psychological and somatic distress in people's experience. Possibly, there is an association between a tendency to invoke psychological explanations and multifactorial explanatory models for somatic symptoms and general beliefs about the body–mind relation. Such explanatory schemas, thus, were more common among women than men in this sample.

REFERENCES

Blaxter, M. (1983). The causes of disease: Women talking. *Social Science & Medicine, 17,* 59–69.
Blaxter, M. (1990). *Health and lifestyles.* London: Routledge.
Folkhälsorapport. (1999). Folkhälsorapport: Om hälsoutvecklingen i Stockholms län. [Public health report: About health development in Stockholm county]. Samhällsmedicin. Stockholms läns landsting. Stockholm: Litohuset.
Gijsbers Van Wijk, C. M., Van-Vliet, K., Kolk, A. M., & Everaerd, W. (1991). Symptom sensitivity and sex differences in physical morbidity: A review of health surveys in the United States and the Netherlands. *Women and Health, 17,* 91–124.
Lundberg, U. (1996). Influence of paid and unpaid work on psychophysiological stress responses of men and women. *Journal of Occupational Health Psychology, 1,* 117–130.
Lundberg, U., Mårdberg, B., & Frankenhauser, M. (1994). The total workload of male and female White-collar workers as related to age, occupational level, and number of children. *Scandinavian Journal of Psychology, 35,* 315–327.

Robbins, J. M., & Kirmayer, L. J. (1991). Attributions of common somatic symptoms. *Psychological Medicine, 21,* 1029–1045.

Verbrugge, L. (1985). Gender and health: An update on hypotheses and evidence. *Journal of Health and Social Behavior, 26,* 156–182.

Verbrugge, L. (1989). The twain meet: Empirical explanations of sex differences in health and mortality. *Journal of Health and Social Behavior, 30,* 282–304.

Walters, V. (1993). Stress, anxiety, and depression: Women's accounts of their health problems. *Social Science & Medicine, 36,* 393–402.

Printed and bound by CPI Group (UK) Ltd, Croydon, CR0 4YY

17/10/2024

01775683-0018